Workbook for
Nursing Assisting
A Foundation in Caregiving

FIFTH EDITION

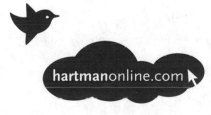

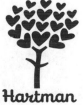

Credits

Managing Editor
Susan Alvare Hedman

Cover Designer
Kirsten Browne

Cover Illustrator
Iveta Vaicule

Production
Elena Reznikova

Proofreaders
Sara Alexander
Joanna Owusu
Jeff Rubin

Copyright Information

Notice to Readers

Though the guidelines and procedures contained in this text are based on consultations with healthcare professionals, they should not be considered absolute recommendations. The instructor and readers should follow employer, local, state, and federal guidelines concerning healthcare practices. These guidelines change, and it is the reader's responsibility to be aware of these changes and of the policies and procedures of her or his healthcare facility.

The publisher, author, editors, and reviewers cannot accept any responsibility for errors or omissions or for any consequences from application of the information in this book and make no warranty, express or implied, with respect to the contents of the book. The publisher does not warrant or guarantee any of the products described herein or perform any analysis in connection with any of the product information contained herein.

Gender Usage

This workbook uses gender pronouns interchangeably to denote healthcare team members and residents.

Table of Contents

Preface

Welcome to the *Workbook for Nursing Assisting: A Foundation in Caregiving*! This workbook is designed to help you review what you have learned from reading your textbook. For this reason, the workbook is organized around learning objectives, just like the textbook and your instructor's teaching material.

These learning objectives work as a built-in study guide. After completing the exercises for each learning objective in the workbook, ask yourself if you can *do* what that learning objective describes.

If you can, move on to the next learning objective. If you cannot, just go back to the textbook, reread that learning objective, and try again.

We have provided procedure checklists at the end of the workbook. There is also a practice test for the certification exam. The answers to the workbook exercises are in your instructor's teaching guide.

Happy learning!

1

The Nursing Assistant in Long-Term Care

1. Review the key terms in Learning Objective 1 before completing the workbook exercises

2. Describe healthcare settings

Multiple Choice
Circle the letter of the answer that best completes the statement or answers the question.

1. Another name for a long-term care facility is a(n)
   (A) Nursing home
   (B) Home health facility
   (C) Assisted living facility
   (D) Adult day services apartment

2. A person who lives in a long-term care facility is called a *resident* because
   (A) The facility is her home
   (B) She is picked up at the end of each day to go home
   (C) She does not have any living family members
   (D) She does not need skilled care

3. Assisted living facilities are usually for
   (A) Residents who need around-the-clock intensive care
   (B) Residents who are generally independent and do not need skilled care
   (C) Residents who will die within six months
   (D) Residents who require acute care

4. How does home health aide care differ from nursing assistant care?
   (A) Home health aides do not assist with personal care.
   (B) Home health aides may clean the home and do laundry.
   (C) Home health aides do not have supervisors.
   (D) Home health care takes place in a hospital, rather than in a long-term care facility.

5. A program of care given by a specialist or a team of specialists to restore or improve function after an illness or injury is called
   (A) Acute care
   (B) Subacute care
   (C) Rehabilitation
   (D) Hospice care

6. Intergenerational care is
   (A) People of the same generation spending time together
   (B) Pets brought into a long-term care facility to help brighten a resident's day
   (C) Elderly adults and children together in the same care setting
   (D) The generation caring for children and aging parents at the same time

3. Explain Medicare and Medicaid

True or False
Mark each statement with either a T for true or an F for false.

1. _____ Medicare is a health insurance program for people who are 65 years of age or older.

2. ____ No one younger than 65 is covered by Medicare.

3. ____ Medicare will pay for any services requested by the resident.

4. ____ A person with limited income might qualify for Medicaid.

5. ____ Medicare and Medicaid pay a fixed amount for services based on residents' needs.

4. Describe the residents in long-term care facilities

True or False

1. ____ It is more important for nursing assistants to know each resident individually than to know general facts about most residents.

2. ____ Most residents living in long-term care facilities are male.

3. ____ Residents with the longest average stay in a healthcare facility are residents admitted for terminal care.

4. ____ Dementia is not a common cause of admission to a long-term care facility.

5. ____ Poor health is not the only reason residents are admitted to long-term care facilities. Often they are admitted due to lack of a support system.

6. ____ Lack of outside support is one reason to care for the whole person instead of only the illness or disease.

5. Describe the nursing assistant's role

Short Answer
Answer each of the following questions in the space provided.

1. What are activities of daily living (ADLs)?

_____

_____

_____

_____

2. Think of one task that might be assigned to a nursing assistant that is not mentioned in the book.

_____

_____

_____

_____

_____

3. Look at the tasks commonly performed by nursing assistants. Which task do you think you will enjoy the most? Which do you think will be the most difficult for you?

_____

_____

_____

_____

_____

_____

_____

_____

_____

_____

6. Discuss professionalism and list examples of professional behavior

Multiple Choice

1. Which of the following best shows professionalism by a nursing assistant?
   (A) A nursing assistant arrives late for her shift, knowing her coworkers can cover for her.
   (B) A nursing assistant takes time to document carefully.
   (C) A nursing assistant uses profanity sometimes, but only if a resident does it first.
   (D) A nursing assistant accepts a tip from a resident's son for taking care of his mother.

2. Takeisha is a new nursing assistant at Parkwood Skilled Nursing Care and wants to make a positive first impression. Which of the following would be the best way for Takeisha to demonstrate professionalism at her new job?
   - (A) She can avoid asking questions so as not to bother her supervisors.
   - (B) She can tell a resident about another resident's condition in order to gain the resident's trust.
   - (C) She can avoid unnecessary work absences.
   - (D) She can address residents by using affectionate nicknames like "Sweetie."

7. List qualities that nursing assistants must have

Scenarios
Read each of the following scenarios and answer the questions that follow.

Nursing assistant Constance Wong is late for five shifts in a row. On the fifth day, her supervisor asks her about this. Constance replies, "It's not my fault. Traffic has been horrible, and I have to drive a long time to get to work."

1. How could Constance have been more humble and open to growth?

   _____
   _____
   _____
   _____
   _____
   _____

Nurse Frederico Gonzalez tells nursing assistant Mary Lupko about a resident's diagnosis of a sexually transmitted infection. He gives specific instructions about the resident's care. Mary sees a fellow nursing assistant across the hall, and says, "How did Joann Timbly get an STI? Her husband hasn't visited in months."

2. How could Mary have been more trustworthy?

   _____
   _____
   _____
   _____
   _____

Nursing assistant DeShawn Brown is tidying Ms. Lee's room. He notices a Buddha statue and asks, "I'm a Christian. Why don't you believe in Jesus?"

3. How could DeShawn have acted in a courteous and respectful manner?

   _____
   _____
   _____
   _____
   _____

Resident Hannah Stein is dying. She tells nursing assistant Mariana Lopez that she always wanted to be nicer to her son and to have a better relationship. Mariana replies, "Well my son won't even talk to me because I wouldn't let him go to a basketball game on a school night." Then Mariana proceeds to tell Mrs. Stein about her divorce and how her son's father never helps out.

4. How could Mariana have been more empathetic?

   _____
   _____
   _____
   _____
   _____
   _____
   _____

Nursing assistant Doug Albin is helping resident Sam Perkins to the bathroom. Sam walks slowly and has to rely on his walker for help. Doug notices that his shift is over in five minutes and says, "Can you walk a little faster? I'm leaving in five minutes!"

5.　How could Doug have been more patient and understanding?

_____
_____
_____
_____
_____
_____
_____
_____

Nursing assistant Wayne Leach just found out his facility is short-staffed tonight, and he will have to help five additional residents get ready for bed. "Oh great," he says. "Now I'll never get this done!"

6.　How could Wayne have been more enthusiastic?

_____
_____
_____
_____
_____
_____
_____
_____

Nurse Aliyah Williams tells nursing assistant Sandra Levy a list of things she wants done. Sandra says she will do them, but when she turns the corner, she forgets what Nurse Williams wanted her to do first. "Oh well," she shrugs. "I'm sure it's not the end of the world."

7.　How could Sandra have been more dependable?

_____
_____
_____
_____
_____
_____
_____
_____
_____
_____
_____
_____

Nursing assistant Tracy Fleming is assigned to help Mr. Ming eat his dinner. Even though she has never met Mr. Ming, she complains, "I can never understand anything these kinds of residents are saying."

8.　How could Tracy have been more unprejudiced?

_____
_____
_____
_____
_____
_____

8. Discuss proper grooming guidelines

Multiple Choice

1. How often should a nursing assistant bathe?
   (A) Several times per week
   (B) Every day
   (C) Every other day
   (D) Twice per week

2. Which of the following should a nursing assistant wear to work?
   (A) A watch
   (B) Bangle bracelets
   (C) A nose ring
   (D) Perfume

3. Which of the following should a nursing assistant wear to work?
   (A) Hoop earrings
   (B) An identification badge
   (C) Acrylic nails
   (D) Aftershave lotion

4. Which of the following is part of proper grooming for a nursing assistant?
   (A) Hair that is tied back
   (B) Long, loose hair
   (C) Long, clean nails
   (D) Dramatic eye makeup

5. Which of the following is true of fingernails?
   (A) Gel nails are the best kind of nails for nursing assistants to wear to work.
   (B) Acrylic nails are the best kind of nails for nursing assistants to wear to work.
   (C) Short, smooth natural nails are the best kind of nails for nursing assistants to wear to work.
   (D) Long, polished nails are the best kind of nails for nursing assistants to wear to work.

9. Define the role of each member of the care team

Matching
Use each letter only once.

1. ____ Activities Director

2. ____ Medical Social Worker (MSW)

3. ____ Nurse (RN)

4. ____ Nursing Assistant (NA)

5. ____ Occupational Therapist (OT or OTD)

6. ____ Physical Therapist (PT or DPT)

7. ____ Physician or Doctor (MD or DO)

8. ____ Physician Assistant (PA)

9. ____ Registered Dietitian Nutritionist (RDN)

10. ____ Resident

11. ____ Respiratory Therapist (RT)

12. ____ Speech-Language Pathologist (SLP)

(A) Determines residents' social needs and helps them get support services, such as counseling or financial assistance

(B) Person whom the care team revolves around

(C) Administers therapy in the form of heat, cold, massage, ultrasound, electrical stimulation, and exercise to muscles, bones, and joints

(D) Performs assigned tasks, such as bathing residents and assisting with elimination, and has the most direct contact with residents

(E) Teaches exercises to help residents improve or overcome speech problems and evaluates ability to swallow food and drink

(F) Assesses residents, creates care plans, monitors progress, and provides treatments and medication

(G) Diagnoses disease or disability and prescribes treatment

(H) Assesses the resident's nutritional status and plans a program of nutritional care

(I) Evaluates a resident's ability to do activities of daily living and develops a treatment plan to help him adapt to disabilities

(J) Plans activities for residents to help them socialize and stay physically and mentally active

(K) Works under the supervision of a doctor and is able to diagnose disease and prescribe treatment and medications

(L) Provides care for people who have respiratory diseases or illnesses

10. Discuss the facility chain of command

Fill in the Blank
Fill in the correct word in each blank below.

1. The chain of command describes the line of

   _____

   in a facility.

2. The _____
   will usually be the nursing assistant's immediate supervisor.

3. When a nursing assistant has a problem with another department, it should be reported to an immediate supervisor or the
   _____ nurse.

4. Following the chain of command helps protect staff from
   _____, which is a legal term for being held responsible for harming someone else.

11. Explain *The Five Rights of Delegation*

Short Answer

1. What are three questions nurses consider before delegating a task?

   _____
   _____
   _____
   _____
   _____
   _____
   _____

2. What are three questions nursing assistants should ask themselves before accepting a delegated task?

   _____
   _____
   _____
   _____
   _____
   _____
   _____
   _____
   _____
   _____

3. If a nursing assistant is unsure about a task that is delegated to him, what should he do?

   _____
   _____
   _____
   _____
   _____
   _____
   _____

12. Describe methods of nursing care and discuss person-centered care

Matching
Use each letter only once.

1. _____ Functional nursing

2. _____ Person-centered care

3. _____ Primary nursing

4. _____ Team nursing

(A) Method of care that revolves around the resident and promotes each individual's preferences, choices, dignity, and interests

(B) Method of care in which a nurse acts as the team leader of the group giving care

(C) Method of care in which each member of the care team is given specific tasks to perform for a large number of residents

(D) Method of care in which the registered nurse gives much of the daily care to residents

13. Explain policy and procedure manuals

Fill in the Blank

1. A _____ is a course of action to be taken every time a certain situation occurs.

2. A complete list of every facility policy is found in the _____ _____.

3. A _____ is a specific way of doing something.

4. The exact way to complete every resident procedure is found in the _____ _____.

14. Describe the long-term care survey process

True or False

1. _____ A survey is conducted by a team of professionals to make sure long-term care facilities are following state and federal regulations.

2. _____ If a surveyor asks a nursing assistant a question and the nursing assistant does not know the answer, she should quickly make one up to avoid being cited.

3. _____ Surveyors will interview residents to get their opinions about the care they receive.

4. _____ Membership in the Joint Commission is mandatory for all long-term care facilities.

2

Ethical and Legal Issues

1. Review the key terms in Learning Objective 1 before completing the workbook exercises

2. Define *law*, *ethics*, and *etiquette*

Multiple Choice

1. _____ have to do with the knowledge of right and wrong.
   (A) Ethics
   (B) Civil laws
   (C) Etiquette issues
   (D) Criminal laws

2. Which of the following is a law?
   (A) A nursing assistant must not gossip about residents or other staff members.
   (B) A nursing assistant must be polite when answering the telephone.
   (C) A nursing assistant must not steal residents' belongings.
   (D) A nursing assistant must not discuss personal problems with coworkers.

3. Laws to protect individuals from people or organizations that try to harm them are
   (A) Civil laws
   (B) Criminal laws
   (C) Felonies
   (D) Misdemeanors

4. A code of courtesy and proper behavior in a certain setting is called
   (A) Civil law
   (B) Criminal law
   (C) Ethics
   (D) Etiquette

3. Discuss examples of ethical and professional behavior

Crossword Puzzle

Across

1. Treating residents with this means allowing them to believe or act as they wish

2. Being able to share in and understand the feelings of others

5. Another word for private

6. Nursing assistants must refuse these when they are offered

Down

1. If a nursing assistant makes a mistake, it is important to do this immediately

3. Being this way means that a nursing assistant is able to speak and act without offending others

4. Ways that a nursing assistant can demonstrate being _____ include being truthful when reporting hours and documenting care accurately

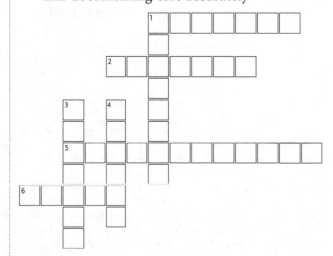

Name: _____

4. Describe a nursing assistant code of ethics

Short Answer

1. What idea do most codes of ethics revolve around?

   _____
   _____
   _____
   _____
   _____
   _____
   _____

2. What is one way for a nursing assistant to help preserve resident safety?

   _____
   _____
   _____
   _____
   _____
   _____
   _____
   _____
   _____

3. If a nursing assistant suspects that a resident is being abused, what should she do?

   _____
   _____
   _____
   _____
   _____
   _____
   _____

5. Explain OBRA

Multiple Choice

1. Why was OBRA (Omnibus Budget Reconciliation Act) passed in 1987?
   (A) As a response to reports of poor care and abuse in long-term care facilities
   (B) Because of complaints of uncooperative residents by nursing assistants
   (C) To control costs in long-term care facilities
   (D) Because most long-term care facilities employed too many nursing assistants

2. How does the OBRA law relate to nursing assistants?
   (A) OBRA tests nursing assistants' knowledge of care procedures.
   (B) OBRA sets minimum requirements for training, competency exams, and in-service education.
   (C) OBRA outlines specific steps for handling infectious material.
   (D) OBRA details how the chain of command works in long-term care facilities.

3. According to OBRA requirements, how many hours of training must nursing assistants complete before being able to be employed?
   (A) 30 hours
   (B) 50 hours
   (C) 75 hours
   (D) 100 hours

4. Which of the following is a part of OBRA's regulations?
   (A) OBRA establishes the correct steps to follow if a nursing assistant is exposed to a bloodborne pathogen.
   (B) OBRA sets the minimum amount that nursing assistants can be paid per hour.
   (C) OBRA details the safe use and hazards of chemicals.
   (D) OBRA requires that states keep a current list of nursing assistants in a state registry.

6. Explain Residents' Rights

Short Answer

For each of the following Residents' Rights, give one example of how a nursing assistant can respect that right.

1. The right to the best quality of life possible

_____

_____

_____

_____

_____

2. The right to receive the correct care in the form of services and activities to maintain a high level of wellness

_____

_____

_____

_____

3. The right to be fully informed about rights and services

_____

_____

_____

_____

4. The right to participate in their own care

_____

_____

_____

_____

5. The right to make independent choices

_____

_____

_____

_____

_____

6. The right to privacy and confidentiality

_____

_____

_____

_____

_____

7. The right to dignity, respect, and freedom

_____

_____

_____

_____

_____

8. The right to security of possessions

_____

_____

_____

_____

Ethical and Legal Issues

9. Rights during transfers and discharges

_____

_____

_____

_____

_____

10. The right to complain

_____

_____

_____

_____

_____

11. The right to visits

_____

_____

_____

_____

_____

_____

12. Rights with regard to social services

_____

_____

_____

_____

_____

_____

7. Explain types of abuse and neglect

Matching
Use each letter only once.

1. ____ Abuse

2. ____ Assault

3. ____ Battery

4. ____ Defamation

5. ____ Domestic violence

6. ____ False imprisonment

7. ____ Financial abuse

8. ____ Involuntary seclusion

9. ____ Libel

10. ____ Malpractice

11. ____ Neglect

12. ____ Negligence

13. ____ Physical abuse

14. ____ Psychological abuse

15. ____ Sexual abuse

16. ____ Sexual harassment

17. ____ Slander

18. ____ Substance abuse

19. ____ Verbal abuse

20. ____ Workplace violence

(A) Actions, or the failure to act or provide proper care for a person, resulting in unintended injury

(B) The repeated use of legal or illegal drugs, cigarettes, or alcohol in a way that is harmful to oneself or others

(C) Any unwelcome sexual advance or behavior that creates an intimidating, hostile, or offensive working environment

(D) Failure to provide needed care, resulting in physical, mental, or emotional harm to a person

(E) The separation of a person from others against the person's will

(F) Unlawful restraint that affects a person's freedom of movement

(G) Verbal, physical, or sexual abuse of staff by other staff members, residents, or visitors

(H) The intentional touching of a person without his or her consent

(I) A threat to harm a person, resulting in the person feeling fearful that he or she will be harmed

(J) Improper or illegal use of a person's money, possessions, property, or other assets

(K) Any statement that is not true that injures a person's reputation

(L) The forcing of unwanted sexual acts or behavior on a person

(M) The use of language that threatens, embarrasses, or insults a person

(N) Emotional harm caused by threatening, frightening, isolating, intimidating, humiliating, or insulting a person

(O) Physical, sexual, or emotional abuse by spouses, intimate partners, or family members

(P) Purposeful mistreatment that causes physical, mental, emotional, or financial pain or injury to a person

(Q) Any treatment, intentional or unintentional, that causes harm to a person's body

(R) Defamation in written form

(S) Defamation in oral form

(T) Professional misconduct that results in damage or injury to a person

Multiple Choice

1. What should a nursing assistant do if he sees or suspects that a resident is being abused?
   (A) The NA should report it to the supervisor and document it at once.
   (B) The NA should keep watching the resident until he is sure he is correct.
   (C) The NA should ignore it unless the resident complains about it.
   (D) The NA should confront the abuser immediately.

2. If a resident wants to make a complaint of abuse, the nursing assistant's responsibility is to
   (A) Investigate that the abuse has really occurred
   (B) Assist the resident in every possible way
   (C) Counsel the resident to help him or her get over the abuse
   (D) Ask other residents if they have seen any abuse occurring

3. An example of sexual abuse is
   (A) A nursing assistant ignores a resident's call light
   (B) A nursing assistant shows a resident a pornographic magazine
   (C) A nursing assistant leaves a resident alone in his room and does not check on him
   (D) A nursing assistant screams at a resident

4. An example of financial abuse is
   (A) A nursing assistant loudly announces in the hallway that a resident has "wet his bed again"
   (B) A nursing assistant makes fun of a resident's religion
   (C) A nursing assistant receives money from a resident to get a faster response time when the resident calls
   (D) A nursing assistant hits a resident when the resident yells at him

5. An example of psychological abuse is
   (A) A nursing assistant pushes a resident to get to the bathroom more quickly
   (B) A nursing assistant tells a resident he needs money for school
   (C) A nursing assistant forces a resident to rub up against her
   (D) While giving care to a resident, a nursing assistant tells him he smells bad

8. Recognize signs and symptoms of abuse and neglect

True or False

1. _____ Ignoring a call light is not considered abuse or neglect.

2. _____ Broken bones, burns, and bruising are all possible signs of abuse.

3. _____ Weight loss can be a sign of neglect.

4. _____ Similar injuries that occur repeatedly probably just mean that the resident is clumsy.

5. _____ If a resident shows fear or anxiety when a certain caregiver is present, this may be a sign of abuse.

6. _____ Mood swings and depression are always caused by illness or chemical imbalance.

7. _____ If a resident is not clean or smells like urine, it probably just means he does not like to bathe.

8. _____ Pressure injuries on a resident's body can indicate neglect.

9. _____ If a resident's family is concerned that abuse is occurring, it is considered a possible sign of abuse.

10. _____ If a nursing assistant only suspects abuse, she should wait until she is sure it is happening before reporting it.

9. Describe the steps taken if a nursing assistant is suspected of abuse

Multiple Choice

1. What is the first thing that normally happens when a report of nursing assistant abuse has been made?
   (A) The NA is fired.
   (B) The NA is suspended.
   (C) The NA is taken into custody.
   (D) The NA is transferred to another facility until the investigation is completed.

2. Which of the following is a step taken after a claim of abuse against a nursing assistant has been made?
   (A) An investigation is performed.
   (B) The nursing assistant is charged with a crime.
   (C) The resident is relocated to another facility.
   (D) The facility is closed to the public.

3. If the claim of abuse is proven to be true, what happens?
   (A) The NA is placed in the abuse registry in addition to other possible penalties.
   (B) The resident is moved to another facility.
   (C) The NA is transferred to another facility in another state.
   (D) The facility is cited for negligence.

10. Discuss the ombudsman's role

Short Answer

1. What is the role of an ombudsman?

_____

_____

_____

_____

_____

_____

_____

_____

_____

2. Which other people or organizations can a resident or his family contact for help or to make a complaint?

_____

_____

_____

_____

_____

_____

_____

_____

11. Explain HIPAA and related terms

Multiple Choice

1. Why was the Health Insurance Portability and Accountability Act (HIPAA) passed?
   (A) To protect the privacy of health information
   (B) To reduce instances of abuse in facilities
   (C) To address infection prevention issues in facilities
   (D) To ensure that elderly people have health insurance

2. What is included under a person's private health information (PHI)?
   (A) The person's activity preferences
   (B) The person's social security number
   (C) The person's favorite food
   (D) The person's favorite color

3. If someone who is not directly involved with a resident's care asks for a resident's PHI, how should the nursing assistant respond?
   (A) The NA should report the request to the resident.
   (B) The NA should ask the resident's family if it is okay to share the information.
   (C) The NA should tell them that the information is confidential and cannot be given.
   (D) The NA should give the person the information.

4. Which of the following is a way to keep private health information confidential?
   (A) Discussing a resident's care with a coworker in a restaurant
   (B) Posting information on Twitter
   (C) Only discussing residents with family or friends
   (D) Logging out or exiting the web browser when finished with computer work

5. Which of the following is considered an invasion of a resident's privacy?
   (A) A nursing assistant tells her supervisor that she thinks a resident is starting to develop a pressure injury.
   (B) A nursing assistant shows her husband a photo of a new resident in her care.
   (C) A nursing assistant documents a resident's complaint of pain.
   (D) A nursing assistant refuses to share information about a resident with the resident's sister.

6. The abbreviation for a law that was enacted as a part of the American Recovery and Reinvestment Act of 2009 and helps expand the protection and security of consumers' electronic health records (EHR) is called
   (A) HISEAL
   (B) HITECH
   (C) HIHELP
   (D) HIQUIET

12. Discuss the Patient Self-Determination Act (PSDA) and advance directives

True or False

1. ____ A DNR order tells healthcare professionals to keep trying to resuscitate a resident in the event of cardiac arrest.

2. ____ The Patient Self-Determination Act is meant to encourage people to make decisions about advance directives.

3. ____ Advance directives designate the kind of care people want in the event they are unable to make those decisions themselves.

4. _____ A living will designates the people who will inherit the resident's estate when he or she dies.

5. _____ A durable power of attorney for health care appoints a person to make medical decisions for a resident in the event he or she becomes unable to do so.

6. _____ Facilities are required by Medicare and Medicaid to give residents and staff information about rights relating to advance directives.

3

Communication Skills

1. Review the key terms in Learning Objective 1 before completing the workbook exercises

2. Explain types of communication

True or False

1. ____ People communicate with words, pictures, and behavior.

2. ____ The receiver and sender do not switch roles as they communicate.

3. ____ Speaking and writing are two examples of verbal communication.

4. ____ How a person's voice sounds and the words he chooses are not important during communication.

5. ____ Nonverbal communication includes posture and facial expressions.

6. ____ Making positive changes in body language will improve communication.

7. ____ A nursing assistant can be helpful by finishing a resident's sentences to show that she understands what he is telling her.

8. ____ The nursing assistant should use mostly facts when communicating with the care team.

Short Answer
State whether each behavior is an example of positive or negative nonverbal communication. Write P for positive or N for negative.

1. ____ Smiling

2. ____ Crossing arms in front of the body

3. ____ Looking away while someone is talking

4. ____ Leaning forward in a chair

5. ____ Pointing at someone while speaking

6. ____ Rolling eyes

7. ____ Tapping a foot

8. ____ Nodding while a person is speaking

3. Explain barriers to communication

Scenarios
Read the scenarios below and answer the questions.

Nursing assistant Barbara Smith thinks resident Mrs. Gold is in pain. Barbara asks her if she is okay. Before Mrs. Gold answers, Barbara looks around the room and begins to gather her supplies to leave. Mrs. Gold simply says, "Yes."

1. Identify the barrier to communication occurring here and suggest a way to avoid it.

   _____

   _____

   _____

   _____

   _____

   _____

   _____

   _____

   _____

   _____

Resident Marla Gibson had a stroke that affects her speech. She asks her nursing assistant for a glass of water. The nursing assistant replies, "I'm not sure where your daughter is," and leaves the room.

2. Identify the barrier to communication occurring here and suggest a way to avoid it.

_____

_____

_____

_____

_____

_____

_____

_____

Nursing assistant Kena Wright asks resident Josiah Crane, "You are NWB, right?" He nods. She reports to the nurse, who says, "That is not true. He is allowed to bear full weight on both legs."

3. Identify the barrier to communication occurring here and suggest a way to avoid it.

_____

_____

_____

_____

_____

_____

_____

_____

_____

_____

Nursing assistant LaShawn Wells sees that resident Eli Levine is having difficulty moving his leg after his total hip replacement surgery. LaShawn says, "I've helped many residents after this type of surgery. You should start doing exercises right away and begin bearing as much weight as possible." Mr. Levine attempts to stand on his leg and yells in pain.

4. Identify the barrier to communication occurring here and suggest a way to avoid it.

_____

_____

_____

_____

_____

_____

_____

_____

Resident Raul Martinez is at risk for dehydration. Nursing assistants are asked to encourage him to drink as much as possible. To find out what Mr. Martinez likes to drink, nursing assistant Gracie Truman asks him, "Do you like orange juice?" He says, "No."

5. Identify the barrier to communication occurring here and suggest a way to avoid it.

_____

_____

_____

_____

_____

_____

_____

_____

_____

_____

Nursing assistant Lyla Cooper is helping resident Josie Bayer get ready to attend a guest lecture with another resident. Josie says, "I don't want to go with her." Lyla asks, "Why not?" Josie replies, "I just don't."

6. Identify the barrier to communication occurring here and suggest a way to avoid it.

_____
_____
_____
_____
_____
_____
_____
_____

Nursing assistant Rashida Fleming is assigned to give a bed bath to Mr. Perez, who speaks very little English. She explains the procedure, and Mr. Perez nods even though he looks a little confused. When she starts to take off his shirt, he gets very upset.

7. Identify the barrier to communication occurring here and suggest a way to avoid it.

_____
_____
_____
_____
_____
_____
_____
_____

4. List ways that cultures impact communication

Multiple Choice

1. Which of the following is true of cultures?
   (A) There are only a few cultures in the world.
   (B) The use of touch is the same for all cultures.
   (C) A culture is a set of learned beliefs, values, and behaviors.
   (D) The use of eye contact is the same for all cultures.

2. If a resident seems to be sensitive to eye contact or touch, a nursing assistant should
   (A) Make eye contact and touch him as much as possible so that the resident is able to get used to it
   (B) Respect his wishes and limit eye contact and touch as much as possible
   (C) Explain to the resident that in the United States things are done differently and he should start adapting
   (D) Ignore his sensitivity and use eye contact and touch as with any other resident

3. Which of the following is a type of unacceptable touch by an NA when working with a resident?
   (A) Sitting on the resident's lap
   (B) Cleaning the resident's arm during a bed bath
   (C) Hugging the resident
   (D) Touching the resident's chin while helping him eat

4. One appropriate way for a nursing assistant to deal with a language barrier with a resident is to
   (A) Use an interpreter
   (B) Teach the resident words in the NA's language
   (C) Speak with other staff in the NA's language in front of the resident
   (D) Get someone else to care for the resident

5. Identify the people a nursing assistant communicates with in a facility

True or False

1. _____ When a nursing assistant first greets a resident, he should introduce himself and identify the resident.

2. _____ In the facility, a nursing assistant may communicate by charting or using the call system.

3. _____ If a nursing assistant has performed a procedure for a resident before, she does not need to explain it the next time she does it.

4. _____ Communication with other departments within a facility is not common and is unimportant.

5. _____ One way to let a resident's family know that staff are providing proper care for him is to always answer call lights promptly.

6. _____ Families can provide valuable information about a resident's preferences and history.

7. _____ If a staff member from a doctor's office calls and asks for information about a resident, the nursing assistant should give it to her.

6. Understand basic medical terminology and abbreviations

Matching
For each of the following abbreviations, write the letter of the correct term from the list below. Use each letter only once.

1. _____ ADLs

2. _____ amb

3. _____ BM

4. _____ c/o

5. _____ DNR

6. _____ DX, dx

7. _____ f/u, F/U

8. _____ IV

9. _____ I&O

10. _____ NPO

11. _____ mL

12. _____ prn, PRN

13. _____ ROM

14. _____ v.s., VS

15. _____ w/c, W/C

(A) Diagnosis

(B) Intravenous

(C) Activities of daily living

(D) Nothing by mouth

(E) Bowel movement

(F) Do not resuscitate

(G) Complains of

(H) Range of motion

(I) Vital signs

(J) Wheelchair

(K) As necessary

(L) Intake and output

(M) Milliliter

(N) Follow up

(O) Ambulate

7. Explain how to convert regular time to military time

Short Answer

Convert the following times to military time:

1. 2:10 p.m. _____

2. 4:30 a.m. _____

3. 10:00 a.m. _____

4. 8:25 p.m. _____

Convert the following military times to regular time:

5. 0600 _____

6. 2320 _____

7. 1927 _____

8. 1800 _____

8. Describe a standard resident chart

Multiple Choice

1. When charting, the nursing assistant's role is limited to which of the following?
   (A) Making changes in residents' diets
   (B) Changing medications when current ones are not working
   (C) Gathering information and reporting to the nurse
   (D) Creating a new care plan

2. Which of the following is true of a resident's medical chart?
   (A) The nursing assistant includes her qualifications in the medical chart.
   (B) Nursing assistants write their diagnoses in the medical chart.
   (C) Information about the resident's roommate is included in the medical chart.
   (D) Nurses' notes are included in the medical chart.

9. Explain guidelines for documentation

Multiple Choice

1. If a mistake is made when charting care manually, the best response by the nursing assistant would be to
   (A) Erase what she has written and enter the correct information
   (B) Draw a line through the error and initial and date it
   (C) Use white correction fluid to cross out the error and then initial and date the white area
   (D) Staple a new sheet to the front of the medical chart that has the correct information

2. When is it appropriate for an NA to chart care before it has been done?
   (A) When a resident requests it
   (B) Never
   (C) When the NA will not have time afterward to do it
   (D) When a procedure will take a long time

3. What color of ink is the best choice for documenting by hand?
   (A) Red
   (B) Black
   (C) Blue
   (D) Green

4. Which statement below is an example of a fact?
   (A) Ms. Lopez was grumpy at dinner.
   (B) Ms. Lopez did not like the chicken.
   (C) Ms. Lopez ate all of her vegetables.
   (D) Ms. Lopez became depressed while eating.

10. Describe the use of computers in documentation

Fill in the Blank

1. Computers can easily store information that can be _____ when needed.

2. Using a computer for charting is faster and more _____ than writing by hand.

3. In some facilities a _____ or tablet is moved from room to room to document care.

4. An NA should not share his personal _____ or login IDs with anyone.

5. An NA should _____ or exit the resident's chart when finished.

6. _____ privacy guidelines apply to electronic documentation.

11. Explain the Minimum Data Set (MDS)

Multiple Choice

1. The Minimum Data Set (MDS) was created to
   (A) Give facilities a standardized approach to care
   (B) Give facilities more flexibility in how care is performed
   (C) Improve infection prevention methods in facilities
   (D) Help train nursing assistants how to do particular care procedures

2. For which of the following situations does an MDS need to be completed?
   (A) When a resident leaves the facility
   (B) Once every five years after the first MDS has been completed
   (C) When there have been no major changes in a resident's condition for two weeks
   (D) Within 14 days of a resident's admission

3. What is the nursing assistant's role regarding the MDS?
   (A) Completing the MDS for each resident
   (B) Reminding the nurse when the MDS needs to be done
   (C) Reporting changes in residents' health
   (D) Deciding how to address problems discovered in the assessment

12. Describe how to observe and report accurately

True or False

1. _____ Nursing assistants may notice more changes in residents than other care team members because they spend the most time with residents.

2. _____ Changes in a resident's condition that endanger the resident should be reported right away.

3. _____ Nursing assistants make decisions regarding residents' health.

4. _____ Critical thinking for nursing assistants means making careful observations and reporting problems.

5. _____ A care plan is a plan for each resident that outlines the steps and tasks needed to help the resident achieve her goals of care.

6. _____ Care plans are developed by nursing assistants.

7. _____ Changes in a resident's weight do not need to be reported unless they are over 10 pounds.

Short Answer

For each of the following, decide whether it is an objective observation (you can see, hear, smell, or touch it) or subjective observation (the resident must tell you about it). Write O for objective and S for subjective.

1. _____ Skin rash

2. _____ Crying

3. _____ Rapid pulse

4. _____ Headache

5. _____ Nausea

6. _____ Vomiting

7. _____ Swelling

8. _____ Cloudy urine

9. _____ Wheezing

10. _____ Feeling sad

11. _____ Red area on skin

12. _____ Fever

13. _____ Dizziness

14. _____ Chest pain

15. _____ Toothache

16. _____ Coughing

17. _____ Fruity breath

18. _____ Itchy arm

Short Answer

1. For each of these four senses, list two observations that a nursing assistant might make using that sense.

- Sight

  _____

  _____

  _____

  _____

  _____

- Hearing

  _____

  _____

  _____

  _____

  _____

- Touch

  _____

  _____

  _____

  _____

  _____

- Smell

  _____

  _____

  _____

  _____

  _____

13. Explain the nursing process

Matching
Use each letter only once.

1. ____ Assessment

2. ____ Diagnosis

3. ____ Evaluation

4. ____ Implementation

5. ____ Planning

(A) Setting goals and creating a care plan to meet the resident's needs

(B) Examining carefully to see if goals were met or progress was achieved

(C) Getting information from many sources to identify actual and potential problems

(D) Putting the care plan into action; giving care

(E) Identifying health problems after looking at all of the resident's needs

14. Discuss the nursing assistant's role in care planning and at care conferences

Multiple Choice

1. The purpose of a care conference is to
   (A) Train nursing assistants in new care skills
   (B) Decide how to remove a resident from a facility
   (C) Share information about residents to develop a plan of care
   (D) Orient new residents to the facility

2. What is the nursing assistant's role at a care conference?
   (A) The NA keeps order at the meeting.
   (B) The NA shares observations about the resident.
   (C) The NA suggests any new medications that might be beneficial for the resident.
   (D) The NA explains the care plan to the resident and his family.

3. If a nursing assistant is not sure what to say at a care conference, she should
   (A) Not attend the conference
   (B) Attend the conference but check with the resident's family about what she can share
   (C) Talk to the nurse before the conference to find out what she should say
   (D) Ask other nursing assistants at the meeting what information she should share

15. Describe incident reporting and recording

Multiple Choice

1. Which of the following would be considered an incident?
   (A) A resident is acting withdrawn.
   (B) A resident accuses a staff member of abuse.
   (C) A resident returns from a family outing later than expected.
   (D) A resident tells a staff member that she does not like her roommate.

2. Documenting an incident and the response to the incident is done in a(n)
   (A) Minimum Data Set report
   (B) Flow sheet report
   (C) Incident report
   (D) Sentinel report

3. Which of the following should the NA include when documenting an incident?
   (A) Facts regarding what the NA saw
   (B) Opinions of why the incident occurred
   (C) Suggestions for changes in the resident's care
   (D) Ideas for revising how incident reports are completed

16. Explain proper telephone etiquette

Multiple Choice

1. An example of proper telephone etiquette is
   (A) Immediately putting the caller on hold without asking
   (B) Identifying the facility to the caller
   (C) Letting the caller know when it is not a good time to call
   (D) Giving the caller any information about residents and staff she needs

2. Which of the following is a general rule for telephone use at a facility?
   (A) All facilities allow the use of cell phones at work.
   (B) Staff information can be disclosed to creditors if they call.
   (C) Resident information can be given to anyone who calls and inquires.
   (D) Resident information cannot be given over the phone.

17. Describe the resident call system

Short Answer

1. What is the purpose of the facility call system?

   _____

   _____

   _____

   _____

   _____

   _____

   _____

2. Why is answering a resident's call light promptly so important?

   _____

   _____

   _____

   _____

   _____

   _____

   _____

   _____

18. Describe the nursing assistant's role in change-of-shift reports and rounds

Fill in the Blank

1. Examples of information passed on to the next shift are _____ that occurred, appetite problems, difficulties with urination, complaints of _____, or a change in the ability to _____.

2. At start-of-shift reports, the NA should listen to important information about all of the _____ in the area.

3. Special information shared during a report may include new _____ and transfers or _____ from the facility.

4. Before the end-of-shift report, the NA should tell the nurses about such things as changes in _____ or temperature and skin changes that could signal the start of a _____.

5. Staff members make scheduled visits to a resident's room to assess the resident's needs and discuss the care plan during a method of reporting called _____.

19. List the information found on an assignment sheet

Matching

1. _____ Activities of daily living

2. _____ Code

3. _____ Code status

4. _____ Range of motion

(A) Exercises done to bring joints through a full range of movement

(B) Explains the type of care that should be provided to a resident in the event of a cardiac arrest, other catastrophic organ failure, or terminal illness

(C) Tasks that are done every day

(D) An emergent medical situation in which specially trained responders provide the necessary care

20. Discuss how to organize work and manage time

Multiple Choice

1. To *prioritize* means to
   (A) Provide privacy during care tasks
   (B) Identify and complete the most important task first
   (C) Make changes to a care plan
   (D) Put in a formal request for a day off with a supervisor

2. When making rounds at the beginning of her shift, the NA should
   (A) Look for tasks that the previous NA left undone to report to the charge nurse
   (B) Start with the resident closest to her and complete all tasks on that resident's assignment sheet before moving on to the next room
   (C) Check in on all residents assigned to her, taking care of immediate needs first
   (D) Go to the supply closet and gather all the supplies she is likely to need for the shift

3. The NA should always get help
   (A) For any task she feels she cannot safely complete
   (B) When she wants to leave early
   (C) When a resident is particularly talkative
   (D) For every care task she performs

4. How can an NA make his shift more efficient?
   (A) He can complete the same care task for all of his assigned residents before moving on to the next task.
   (B) He can plan ahead to have all supplies ready for a procedure.
   (C) He can make personal calls on his cell phone as he assists a resident with tasks such as eating.
   (D) He can decide to swap assignments with a coworker based on who is faster at certain tasks.

5. Which of the following can help an NA stay organized?
   (A) The NA can decline to perform any task that is not on her schedule.
   (B) The NA can list reminders about a resident's care needs on a notepad.
   (C) The NA can rely on her memory to remember important tasks.
   (D) The NA can decide which of her assigned tasks to leave for the next shift.

4

Communication Challenges

1. Review the key terms in Learning Objective 1 before completing the workbook exercises

2. Identify communication guidelines for visual impairment

Multiple Choice

1. A partial or complete loss of function or ability is an
   (A) Imperative
   (B) Impairment
   (C) Infraction
   (D) Infinite

2. One disease that can cause visual impairment is
   (A) Diabetes
   (B) Chronic Obstructive Pulmonary Disease
   (C) Dermatitis
   (D) Irritable Bowel Syndrome

3. What is the first step a nursing assistant should take before touching a resident who has a visual impairment?
   (A) The NA should put away the resident's personal items.
   (B) The NA should read the menu.
   (C) The NA should change the resident's sheets.
   (D) The NA should identify herself.

4. What is important for an NA to note about a resident's eyeglasses?
   (A) Whether the eyeglasses are stylish
   (B) Whether the eyeglasses fit properly
   (C) Whether the eyeglasses have glass or plastic lenses
   (D) Whether the lenses darken automatically when exposed to sunlight

5. Which of the following would be the best way for an NA to explain the position of objects to a resident who has a visual impairment?
   (A) The NA can take the resident around the room and have her touch items to know where they are located.
   (B) The NA can let the resident know how far away objects are by using approximate measurements in inches, feet, and yards.
   (C) The NA can describe the position of objects using the face of an imaginary clock.
   (D) The NA can use the directional terms *north*, *south*, *east*, and *west* to describe the position of objects.

3. Identify communication guidelines for hearing impairment

Multiple Choice

1. Which of the following is a symptom of hearing loss?
   (A) Trouble hearing high-pitched noises
   (B) Trouble hearing vowels
   (C) Being able to understand the meanings of words
   (D) Being able to hear people who are outside of the room

2. Which of the following is the best way for a nursing assistant to communicate with a resident who has a hearing impairment?
   (A) The NA should exaggerate the pronunciation of words.
   (B) The NA should shout when speaking.
   (C) The NA should raise the pitch of her voice.
   (D) The NA should use simple words and short sentences.

4. Explain defense mechanisms as methods of coping with stress

True or False

1. ____ Defense mechanisms allow a person to release tension.

2. ____ Repression means seeing feelings in others that are actually feelings within oneself.

3. ____ Displacement means transferring a strong feeling to a less threatening object.

4. ____ Defense mechanisms help a person face the reasons a situation has occurred.

5. ____ Denial is rejecting a thought or feeling.

6. ____ Regression is making excuses to justify something.

5. List communication guidelines for anxiety

Short Answer

1. Define *anxiety*.

_____

_____

_____

_____

2. List four physical symptoms of anxiety.

_____

_____

_____

_____

_____

_____

3. List five guidelines for communicating with a resident who is anxious.

_____

_____

_____

_____

_____

_____

_____

_____

_____

_____

6. Discuss communication guidelines for depression

True or False

1. ____ Losses that a resident may be experiencing include the loss of a spouse, friends, and independence.

2. ____ Major depressive disorder can be managed, but it cannot be cured.

3. ____ One behavior that is associated with major depressive disorder is a lack of interest in activities.

4. ____ Most people who have this mental health disorder could choose to be well if they wanted to.

5. ____ It is never a good idea for a nursing assistant to touch a resident who has depression.

6. ____ NAs should not talk to adults as if they were children.

7. ____ Residents who have major depressive disorder will never want to talk about their feelings.

8. ____ NAs should report possible signs of depression right away.

7. Identify communication guidelines for anger

Fill in the Blank

1. _____
   is a natural emotion that may be expressed by residents, their families and friends, and staff members.

2. Loss of _____
   can cause a resident to be angry.

3. Narrowed _____ and clenched or raised _____
   are signs of anger.

4. Anger may also be expressed by withdrawing or being _____.

5. If a resident becomes angry frequently, a _____ may be scheduled.

6. When dealing with a resident who is angry, the NA should try to find out what _____ the resident's anger.

7. The NA should not _____ with an angry resident.

8. The NA can try to involve the resident in _____.

9. Being _____
   means being confident in dealing with other people. Being _____ means expressing oneself in a way that humiliates or overpowers another person.

8. Identify communication guidelines for combative behavior

Multiple Choice

1. Which of the following would be the best response by a nursing assistant when a resident is being combative?
   (A) The NA should call for the nurse immediately.
   (B) The NA should stay as close to the resident as she can.
   (C) The NA should respond to insults with humor or sarcasm.
   (D) The NA should threaten the resident if the behavior does not stop.

2. A nursing assistant's responsibility when a resident becomes combative is to
   (A) Leave the resident alone until he is calm
   (B) Let the resident know that he is upsetting everyone and needs to stop
   (C) Keep other people at a safe distance
   (D) Restrain the resident if he does not calm down

3. Under what circumstances may a nursing assistant hit a resident?
   (A) Any time a resident becomes combative
   (B) If the resident threatens to hit the nursing assistant first
   (C) Only if the resident actually hits the nursing assistant
   (D) Never

9. Identify communication guidelines for inappropriate sexual behavior

Crossword Puzzle

Across

2. Nursing assistants must not do this regarding residents' sexual behavior

5. A nursing assistant should not _____
   when encountering an embarrassing situation, but instead should remain professional and calm.

6. Touching or rubbing sexual organs in order to give oneself or another person sexual pleasure

Down

1. Removing these in public areas is one example of inappropriate sexual behavior

3. One illness that can cause inappropriate sexual behavior

4. What a nursing assistant should provide if she witnesses consenting adults in a sexual situation

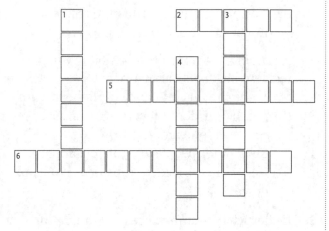

10. Identify communication guidelines for disorientation and confusion

Short Answer

1. Define *disorientation* and *confusion*.

_____

_____

_____

_____

_____

_____

_____

_____

2. List three things that a resident who is oriented should be able to tell the nursing assistant.

_____

_____

_____

_____

_____

_____

_____

_____

_____

3. Name five physical problems that may cause confusion.

_____

_____

_____

_____

_____

_____

_____

_____

_____

_____

_____

4. How can a nursing assistant make tasks easier for a person who is disoriented or confused?

_____

_____

_____

_____

_____

_____

_____

_____

11. Identify communication guidelines for a resident who is comatose

Multiple Choice

1. Which of the following is true of a resident who is comatose?
   (A) A resident who is comatose is conscious.
   (B) A resident who is comatose can respond to changes in the environment.
   (C) A resident who is comatose may be able to hear what is going on in the room.
   (D) A nursing assistant should avoid speaking to a resident who is comatose.

2. Which of the following should a nursing assistant do when caring for a resident who is comatose?
   (A) The NA should explain each procedure that he will be performing to the resident.
   (B) The NA should avoid announcing when he enters and leaves the room since the resident is not aware of anything.
   (C) The NA should remain silent at all times to avoid disturbing the resident.
   (D) The NA should not touch the resident.

12. Identify communication guidelines for functional barriers

Fill in the Blank

1. Some things that can interfere with the ability to speak include difficulty _____, physical problems with the _____ or _____, or an artificial _____.

2. Birth defects such as a cleft _____ may make speech difficult.

3. A(n) _____ is an opening through the neck into the trachea that is surgically created.

4. The resident can _____ anything that is not understood by the NA.

5. The NA should not remove a resident's _____ for any reason.

6. The NA should always report if the resident has poorly fitting

   _____.

7. The NA should be _____ to the resident's situation by imagining how it might feel to have a tube in the nose, mouth, or throat.

5

Diversity and Human Needs and Development

1. Review the key terms in Learning Objective 1 before completing the workbook exercises

2. Explain health and wellness

Multiple Choice

1. The focus of health should be
   (A) On the whole person
   (B) On the person's diagnosed disease
   (C) On the person's disability
   (D) On the person's poor health habits

2. The types of wellness are
   (A) Physical, social, emotional, intellectual, and ethical
   (B) Physical, social, emotional, financial, and spiritual
   (C) Physical, social, sexual, intellectual, and nutritional
   (D) Physical, social, emotional, intellectual, and spiritual

3. Explain the importance of holistic health care

Multiple Choice

1. Holistic health care involves
   (A) Dividing a system into parts
   (B) Caring only for a person's physical needs
   (C) Caring only for a person's psychosocial needs
   (D) Caring for the whole person

2. Which of the following is an example of a psychosocial need?
   (A) Need for food
   (B) Need to nurture spirituality
   (C) Need to be free from pain
   (D) Need for shelter

3. Which of the following is an example of giving holistic care to a resident?
   (A) Asking a resident to talk about her day while giving her a bath
   (B) Rushing a resident through dinner to get tasks done more quickly
   (C) Choosing a resident's clothes for him so he does not have to worry about it
   (D) Trying to convert a resident to the nursing assistant's religion so that they will have something in common

4. Identify basic human needs and discuss Maslow's Hierarchy of Needs

Fill in the Blank

1. A _____ is something necessary for a person to survive and grow.

2. Residents need to feel as if they

   _____

   in their new home.

3. The first needs nursing assistants help residents meet are _____ needs like food and water, rest, and sleep.

4. Moving a person from her home into a facility can cause _____.

5. Residents may feel less of a sense of self-worth as they become

   _____ on others.

6. The highest need a person can achieve, according to Maslow, is _____ _____.

5. Identify ways to accommodate cultural differences

True or False

1. ____ Generally, a nursing assistant will not need to understand different cultures to provide better care to residents.

2. ____ Culture and background do not affect the way people behave when they are ill.

3. ____ A nursing assistant should respond to new ideas with acceptance rather than prejudice.

4. ____ People of all cultures tend to be embarrassed about discussing their health.

5. ____ In the United States, there are only a few different cultures.

6. ____ Cultural competence is an ongoing process of learning about other cultures to provide better care.

6. Discuss the role of the family in health care

Multiple Choice

1. Which of the following is true of families?
    (A) Some families are the right kind of family, while others are the wrong kind.
    (B) Families play an important role in residents' health care.
    (C) Unmarried couples should not be considered a type of family.
    (D) Families should not be allowed privacy for visits with residents.

2. Which of the following is an example of a nuclear family?
    (A) A mother, a father, and a child
    (B) A mother, a father, a grandfather, and a child
    (C) An uncle, a friend, and one parent
    (D) A cousin, an aunt, and a child

3. Which of the following is the best response by the nursing assistant when a resident has his family visiting?
    (A) The NA should do everything possible to help the resident prepare for the visit.
    (B) The NA should ignore the visitors so as not to bother them.
    (C) The NA should tell the resident's family funny stories about the resident.
    (D) The NA should watch the family closely to make sure the resident is not abused during the visit.

7. Explain how to meet emotional needs of residents and their families

Crossword Puzzle

Across

3. Staff members who are prone to this are at risk for inappropriate relationships with residents

4. The care team member that families should be referred to when they ask nursing assistants about a resident's diagnosis

5. Nursing assistants must maintain these when working with residents and their families

6. "Everything will be fine" is an example, as is, "It all works out in the end."

Down

1. Nursing assistants can answer questions asked by residents and their families as long as the questions are within the NA's _____

2. It is important that nursing assistants listen and not do this when residents go to them with their problems

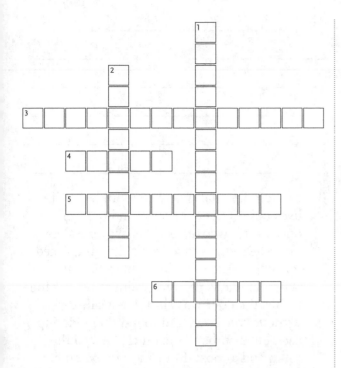

5. ____ Hinduism

6. ____ Islam

7. ____ Judaism

(A) The Five Pillars of this religion include ritual prayer five times daily and donations to the poor and needy

(B) Baptism and communion may be part of this religion's practices

(C) Believe that they do not know or cannot know if God exists

(D) Believe that a person can reach Nirvana, the highest spiritual plane, after traveling through birth, life, and death

(E) Believe that how a person moves toward enlightenment is determined by karma (the result of actions in this life and past lives that can determine one's destiny in future lives)

(F) Believe that God gave them laws and commandments through Moses in the form of the Torah

(G) Actively deny the existence of any deity (higher power)

8. Explain ways to help residents with their spiritual needs

True or False

1. ____ A resident's religious items must be handled carefully

2. ____ Respecting religious beliefs includes letting Muslim residents know about Christianity.

3. ____ Spiritual needs are different for each person.

4. ____ Some people consider themselves spiritual but do not believe in a higher power.

5. ____ Residents who do not believe in God will not feel as strongly about this belief as residents who do.

Matching
Write the letter of the correct description beside each term related to religious faith or belief. Use each letter only once.

1. ____ Agnosticism

2. ____ Atheism

3. ____ Buddhism

4. ____ Christianity

9. Identify ways to accommodate sexual needs

Matching
Use each letter only once.

1. ____ Asexual

2. ____ Bisexual

3. ____ Celibate

4. ____ Coming out

5. ____ Cross-dresser

6. ____ Gay

7. ____ Heterosexual

8. ____ Lesbian

9. ____ LGBTQ

10. ____ Transgender

11. ____ Transition

Name: _____

(A) The process of changing genders, which can include legal procedures and medical measures

(B) A person who abstains from sexual activity

(C) A person whose physical, emotional, and/or romantic attraction is for people of the same sex

(D) Typically a heterosexual man who sometimes wears clothing and other items associated with women

(E) A person whose gender identity conflicts with his or her birth sex

(F) A person whose physical, emotional, and/or romantic attraction is for people of the same gender or a different gender

(G) A person whose physical, emotional, and/or romantic attraction is for people of the opposite sex

(H) Acronym for lesbian, gay, bisexual, transgender, and queer

(I) A woman whose physical, emotional, and/or romantic attraction is for other women

(J) A person who does not experience sexual attraction to any gender

(K) A continual process of revealing one's sexual orientation or gender identity to others

Short Answer

1. Gilda and Samantha both live in a care facility. Gilda is widowed, and Samantha has never been married. They met when Gilda was admitted six months ago. Gilda and Samantha have been sitting at the same table to eat their meals since Gilda moved in. Recently they have started spending time watching TV and playing cards in the day room together. Yesterday they took a walk outside. Linda, a nursing assistant, was gazing out the window and noticed them holding hands. Then she saw them stop behind the building and share a quick kiss. What are some responses that would respect Samantha's and Gilda's dignity and rights?

_____

_____

2. Mr. Ramirez has a private room. His wife lives quite a distance away and only visits once every two weeks. The last time she visited, she requested a dinner tray and asked for both meals to be brought to his room. When Linda went to his room to deliver the meals, the door was shut. She walked in without knocking, and found them kissing each other in bed. She quickly exited the room and almost dropped the food on her way out. What could Linda have done differently? What should she do now that there has been an embarrassing moment?

_____

_____

_____

_____

_____

_____

_____

_____

_____

3. What are two reasons for a lack of sexual expression in long-term care facilities?

_____

_____

_____

_____

_____

10. Describe the stages of human growth and development

Fill in the Blank

1. _____ refers to physical changes that can be measured.

2. _____ means the emotional, social, and physical changes that occur in a person's life.

3. _____ development is the process of gaining an ability to do things like grasp items.

4. _____ development is the process of children forming a sense of right and wrong.

5. _____ development focuses on how children think and learn.

6. _____ development is the process of learning to relate to other people.

7. _____ development has to do with the reproductive changes that occur when young people reach puberty.

Multiple Choice

1. In which stage of development is playing dress-up in parents' clothing common?
   (A) Toddler
   (B) Preschool
   (C) Adolescence
   (D) Infancy

2. Both genders become fully sexually mature during this stage of development:
   (A) School-age
   (B) Adolescence
   (C) Middle adulthood
   (D) Late adulthood

3. Decisions about education, employment, and marriage often occur during this stage:
   (A) Young adulthood
   (B) Preadolescence
   (C) Late adulthood
   (D) Adolescence

4. Which of the following is true of late adulthood?
   (A) People no longer need to stay connected to others.
   (B) People in this stage do not need to remain active.
   (C) People often retire from jobs and may need more medical care.
   (D) People undergo very few changes during this stage of life.

11. Discuss stereotypes of the elderly

Multiple Choice

1. Making a biased generalization based on distorted ideas about a group is
   (A) Stereotyping
   (B) Exaggerating
   (C) Opining
   (D) Discriminating

2. Which of the following is a common stereotype about the elderly?
   (A) Elderly people have sharp memories.
   (B) Elderly people are sexually active.
   (C) Elderly people are less intelligent than younger people.
   (D) Elderly people are very independent.

3. Most older people
   (A) Do not like to leave home
   (B) Are active and have many interests
   (C) Cannot manage their money
   (D) Are ill and dependent

12. Discuss developmental disabilities

True or False

1. ____ Developmental disabilities are present at birth or emerge during childhood, up to age 22.

2. ____ Developmental disabilities cause difficulty with language, learning, and self-care.

3. ____ The most common developmental disability is autism spectrum disorder.

4. ____ People who have developmental disabilities prefer to be treated like children.

5. ____ Developmental disabilities can be cured with medication.

6. ____ An intellectual disability is not the same thing as a mental health disorder.

7. ____ Cerebral palsy generally does not worsen as a person gets older.

8. ____ There are four types of cerebral palsy.

9. ____ A person with a profound degree of intellectual disability will require more care than a person with a severe degree of intellectual disability.

10. ____ The resident and his family should be consulted about which term(s) to use to refer to his disability.

11. ____ Taking folic acid during pregnancy prevents all developmental disabilities.

12. ____ Individuals with intellectual disabilities rarely enjoy social interaction.

13. ____ A person born with spina bifida may experience a combination of different problems with ambulation and learning disabilities.

14. ____ Fragile X syndrome is the name for severe autism spectrum disorder.

15. ____ A person with autism spectrum disorder will usually thrive in new environments.

16. ____ A nursing assistant may need to use alternate methods of communication with residents who cannot speak.

17. ____ Cerebral palsy can be the result of trauma during birth.

18. ____ Autism spectrum disorder affects social and communication skills.

19. ____ Fragile X syndrome can be diagnosed through a blood test.

20. ____ Physical therapy can help residents who have autism spectrum disorder.

21. ____ Residents who have a developmental disability should always have their activities of daily living done for them, rather than doing them independently.

22. ____ A person with an intellectual disability develops at a below-average rate.

23. ____ Special diets may be part of the care plan for a resident with a developmental disability.

24. ____ Focused interests are a common symptom of spina bifida.

6

Infection Prevention and Control

1. Review the key terms in Learning Objective 1 before completing the workbook exercises

2. Define *infection prevention* and discuss types of infections

Matching
Use each letter only once.

1. ____ Communicable disease

2. ____ Cross-infection

3. ____ Healthcare-associated infection (HAI)

4. ____ Infection prevention

5. ____ Localized infection

6. ____ Microorganism

7. ____ Pathogens

8. ____ Reinfection

9. ____ Resistance

10. ____ Systemic infection

(A) A living thing or organism that is so small that it is only visible under a microscope

(B) Infection that is in the bloodstream and is spread throughout the body

(C) The body's ability to prevent infection and disease

(D) Microorganisms that are capable of causing infection and disease

(E) Infection that is limited to a specific location in the body

(F) The physical movement or transfer of harmful bacteria from one person, object, or place to another, or from one part of the body to another

(G) An infectious disease transmissible by direct contact or by indirect contact

(H) Being infected again with the same pathogen

(I) Set of methods used to prevent and control the spread of disease

(J) An infection acquired within a healthcare setting during the delivery of medical care

3. Discuss terms related to infection prevention

True or False

1. ____ Sterilization means all microorganisms are destroyed, including those that form spores.

2. ____ Medical asepsis means that a facility is completely free from all microorganisms.

3. ____ A nursing assistant must wash his hands before leaving a dirty utility room.

4. ____ Transmission is the process of removing pathogens from an object.

5. ____ An object can be called *clean* if it is not contaminated with pathogens.

6. ____ Spore-forming organisms, a special group of organisms that produce a protective covering that is difficult to penetrate, are killed by disinfection.

Name: _____

7. ____ Clean and dirty equipment, linen, and supplies are normally stored in the same utility room.

4. Describe the chain of infection

Short Answer

1. What does the chain of infection describe?

_____

_____

_____

_____

_____

2. How many links in the chain of infection must be broken for infection to be prevented?

_____

_____

3. List the six links of the chain of infection.

_____

_____

_____

_____

_____

_____

5. Explain why the elderly are at a higher risk for infection

Multiple Choice

1. One reason that older people are at a greater risk for acquiring infections is
   (A) Their bones become stronger
   (B) They are hospitalized more often
   (C) They recover more quickly from illness
   (D) Their circulation increases

2. Which of the following is a factor associated with aging that increases the risk of infection?
   (A) Thicker skin
   (B) Increased circulation
   (C) Use of catheters and other tubing
   (D) Increased mobility

6. Describe Centers for Disease Control and Prevention (CDC) and explain Standard Precautions

Fill in the Blank

1. The abbreviation for the government agency that promotes public health and safety and attempts to control and prevent disease is

   _____.

2. The two levels of precautions in the infection prevention system recommended by the CDC are Standard Precautions and

   _____

   _____.

3. Standard Precautions means treating all blood, body fluids, nonintact skin, and mucous membranes as if they were

   _____.

4. An NA cannot tell by looking at residents or even by reading their medical charts if they have a(n)

   _____ disease.

5. An NA should wear a

   _____

   and protective _____
   if there is a chance of coming into contact
   with splashing or spraying body fluids.

6. Razor blades and other sharps should be disposed of in a _____
   container for sharps.

7. An NA should never transfer

   _____ items or any

   kind of _____ from one
   room to another.

8. An NA should never place

   _____ items like
   bedpans on an overbed table.

9. When cleaning anything, the NA should move from the

_____ to the

_____ area.

7. Define *hand hygiene* and identify when to wash hands

True or False

1. _____ Handwashing is the most important way to prevent the spread of disease.

2. _____ Bacteria can be removed from artificial nails with thorough handwashing.

3. _____ The use of hand lotion can prevent skin from cracking.

4. _____ A nursing assistant must wash her hands every time she removes her gloves.

5. _____ A nursing assistant must wash his hands after he blows his nose.

6. _____ A nursing assistant does not need to wash her hands before obtaining clean linen from a cart.

7. _____ When washing hands, the nursing assistant should use friction for no more than five seconds.

8. _____ Using alcohol-based hand rubs means that nursing assistants do not need to wash their hands with soap and water.

8. Discuss the use of personal protective equipment (PPE) in facilities

Multiple Choice

1. Which of the following is the main factor that determines what type of personal protective equipment (PPE) must be worn for a specific task?
   (A) The type of exposure that may be encountered
   (B) The resident's preference on what type of PPE should be worn
   (C) Whether or not specific kinds of PPE are big enough to fit the nursing assistant
   (D) How comfortable the resident's family is with the choice of PPE

2. What step should the nursing assistant take right after she removes and discards PPE??
   (A) Gathering clean PPE for the next task
   (B) Restocking glove boxes
   (C) Performing hand hygiene
   (D) Documenting resident care

3. If a gown becomes wet during care, what should the nursing assistant do?
   (A) Dry it with clean paper towels
   (B) Remove the gown and shake it gently until it air dries
   (C) Spot clean the wet areas with a bleach solution
   (D) Discard it and don a new gown

4. Immediately after giving care, what should the nursing assistant do with his gloves?
   (A) He should wash his gloves.
   (B) He should don a second pair of gloves over the first pair.
   (C) He should remove the gloves and wash his hands.
   (D) He should check the gloves for holes and if they are not torn, he should keep them on for use with the next resident.

5. Which of the following should be worn when it is likely that blood or body fluids may be splashed into the eyes?
   (A) Goggles
   (B) Hat
   (C) Eyeglasses
   (D) Sunglasses

Short Answer

Make a check mark (✓) next to the tasks that require a nursing assistant to wear gloves.

1. _____ Contact with body fluids

2. _____ Hanging laundry

3. _____ When the NA may touch blood

4. _____ Brushing a resident's hair

5. _____ Assisting with perineal care

6. _____ Giving a massage to a resident with acne on his back

7. _____ Hugging a resident

8. _____ Shaving a resident

9. List guidelines for handling linen and equipment

Crossword Puzzle

Across

4. Type of container in which sharps should be disposed

5. Linen should be rolled so that the dirtiest area is here

6. Nursing assistants should not do this to dirty linen or clothes

Down

1. Another word for single-use equipment

2. Must be worn when handling soiled linen

3. Abbreviation for federal government agency that sets guidelines for the storage and disposal of linens and equipment

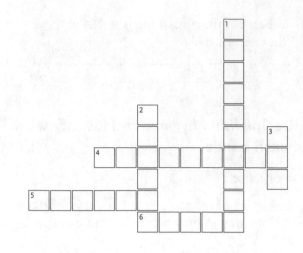

10. Explain how to handle spills

Short Answer

1. Why are spills in a healthcare facility dangerous?

   _____

   _____

   _____

   _____

2. When something is spilled, what is the first step that a nursing assistant should take?

   _____

   _____

   _____

   _____

3. If a nursing assistant spills a substance on her body, what should she do?

   _____

   _____

   _____

   _____

   _____

   _____

11. Discuss Transmission-Based Precautions

Short Answer
Write the first letter of the correct type of precaution (A for Airborne, D for Droplet, or C for Contact) for each of the following.

1. _____ *Clostridioides difficile* (*C. diff*) is an example of an infection requiring these type of precautions.

2. _____ Transmission of a microorganism can occur with direct contact; for example, a nursing assistant bathing a resident.

3. _____ These precautions reduce the risk of spreading tuberculosis.

4. _____ Microorganisms can be spread by talking, singing, sneezing, laughing, breathing, or coughing.

5. _____ Diseases can be transmitted through the air.

6. _____ Infection can be spread by touching contaminated personal items.

12. Describe care of the resident in an isolation unit

Short Answer

1. If it is allowed, why is it important for a nursing assistant to spend as much time as possible with a resident who is in isolation?

_____

_____

_____

_____

_____

2. Which type of supplies are best for residents in isolation?

_____

_____

_____

_____

3. What are items that may be needed when setting up an isolation cart?

_____

_____

_____

_____

_____

_____

_____

_____

13. Explain OSHA's Bloodborne Pathogen Standard

Fill in the Blank

1. _____ is the abbreviation of the government agency that regulates the safety of workers in the United States.

2. The _____ _____ Standard is the law that requires healthcare facilities to protect employees from blood-borne health hazards.

3. A(n) _____ _____ plan outlines specific work practices to pre-vent exposure to infectious material and identifies step-by-step procedures to follow when exposures do occur.

4. In the healthcare setting, contact with _____ or _____ is the most common way to be infected with a bloodborne disease.

5. The employer is responsible for providing a free _____ vaccine to all employees after hire.

14. Discuss two important bloodborne diseases

Multiple Choice

1. How does the human immunodeficiency virus (HIV) cause the body to be unable to fight infection?
   (A) It causes cirrhosis.
   (B) It causes liver cancer.
   (C) It weakens the immune system.
   (D) It poisons the blood.

2. What is one way that HIV is spread?
   (A) By coughing or sneezing
   (B) By using infected needles
   (C) By hugging
   (D) Through handshakes

3. Hepatitis ___ and ___ are bloodborne diseases that can cause death.
   (A) A and B
   (B) B and C
   (C) C and E
   (D) A and C

4. Which of the following statements is true of hepatitis B?
   (A) Hepatitis B is commonly spread by the fecal-oral route.
   (B) There is no vaccine for hepatitis B.
   (C) Hepatitis B can be spread by contact with infected needles.
   (D) Hepatitis B can be spread through contaminated water.

15. Discuss MRSA, VRE, C. difficile, and CRE

True or False

1. ____ Multidrug-resistant organisms (MDROs) are not a serious problem in healthcare facilities.

2. ____ Methicillin-resistant Staphylococcus aureus (MRSA) is mostly spread by direct physical contact with infected people.

3. ____ Proper hand hygiene can help prevent the spread of vancomycin-resistant Enterococcus (VRE).

4. ____ The bacteria enterococci often causes problems in healthy people.

5. ____ Both hand rubs and washing hands with soap and water are considered equally effective when dealing with C. difficile.

6. ____ The overuse of antibiotics may alter the normal intestinal flora and increase the risk of developing C. difficile diarrhea.

7. ____ There is no test that can diagnose C. difficile.

8. ____ Carbapenem-resistant Enterobacteriaceae (CRE) is most often spread through direct contact with an infected person.

9. ____ To help protect against the spread of influenza (the flu), a person should maintain a distance of at least two feet from an infected person.

10. ____ Norovirus is not a type of contagious virus.

7

Safety and Body Mechanics

1. Review the key terms in Learning Objective 1 before completing the workbook exercises

2. List common accidents in facilities and ways to prevent them

True or False

1. _____ An important way that nursing assistants can help prevent falls is to respond to call lights promptly.

2. _____ Wearing long clothing and going without shoes help prevent falls.

3. _____ A nursing assistant must identify each resident before providing care or serving food.

4. _____ Disoriented or confused residents should not be identified before serving food since they do not understand who they are.

5. _____ Burns can cause a rapid deterioration in a resident's condition.

6. _____ In order to help prevent burns, the water temperature should be 130°F when giving a bath.

7. _____ Liquids can cause burns.

8. _____ A resident who is confused may eat hair care products or flowers.

9. _____ To help prevent choking, residents should eat quickly.

10. _____ Sitting up straight while eating helps prevent choking.

11. _____ Large pieces of food are less likely to cause choking.

12. _____ Protecting arms and legs while moving residents helps prevent injury.

13. _____ If an NA needs help lifting a resident but nobody is around, she should lift the resident anyway.

14. _____ If no eye wash station is available after an eye splash, the NA should rinse his eyes immediately with water at a sink.

3. Explain the Safety Data Sheet (SDS)

Short Answer

1. List five examples of information that is found on a Safety Data Sheet (SDS).

_____

_____

_____

_____

_____

_____

_____

2. What are two things that a nursing assistant must know about the SDS?

_____

_____

_____

_____

_____

4. Describe safety guidelines for sharps and biohazard containers

Fill in the Blank

1. The NA should always don
   _____ before
   touching a sharps container.

2. It is important for an NA to keep her hands
   _____ of
   the opening of a biohazard container when
   dropping an object into it.

3. When carrying a sharps container, the NA
   should carry it by the
   _____ of
   the container.

4. Sharps containers should be replaced when
   they are _____
   full (or what facility policy states).

5. Biohazard containers or bags are used to dis-
   pose of items contaminated with infectious
   waste, except for anything
   _____.

5. Explain the principles of body mechanics and apply them to daily activities

Matching
Use each letter only once.

1. ____ Alignment

2. ____ Back and body injuries

3. ____ Base of support

4. ____ Body mechanics

5. ____ Center of gravity

(A) Foundation that supports an object

(B) The point in the body where the most
weight is concentrated

(C) When the two sides of the body are mirror
images of each other

(D) The way the parts of the body work together
when a person moves

(E) Common risks that nursing assistants face
when working in healthcare facilities

Multiple Choice

1. When moving an object, which of the fol-
   lowing is the best place for the nursing
   assistant to stand?
   (A) Close to the object
   (B) A couple of feet behind the object
   (C) To the right of the object
   (D) About 36 inches in front of the object

2. When lifting an object, how should the NA's
   knees be positioned?
   (A) The knees should be locked.
   (B) The knees should be bent.
   (C) The knees should be together.
   (D) The knees should be straight.

3. Objects should be _____ rather than
   lifted.
   (A) Pulled
   (B) Raised
   (C) Pushed
   (D) Carried

6. Define two types of restraints and discuss problems associated with restraints

Multiple Choice

1. What is one reason the use of restraints in
   healthcare facilities has been restricted?
   (A) Restraints are too expensive.
   (B) Restraints were overused by caregivers.
   (C) Training nursing assistants to use
   restraints is too difficult.
   (D) Nursing assistants do not have time to
   monitor residents who are restrained.

2. When may restraints be used?
   (A) For staff convenience
   (B) With a doctor's order
   (C) To discipline residents
   (D) Whenever staff wants to use them

3. Which of the following is a potential effect
   of restraint use?
   (A) Pressure injuries
   (B) Increased blood circulation
   (C) Increased bone mass
   (D) Better sleep habits

7. Discuss restraint alternatives

1. _____
   care means that restraints are not kept or
   used for any reason.

2. Creative ideas that help avoid the use of
   restraints are called _____
   _____.

3. The NA should answer
   _____
   _____
   immediately.

4. The doctor may add
   _____ into
   the care plan.

5. Confused residents should be allowed to
   _____
   in designated safe areas.

6. Visits and _____
   interaction should be increased.

7. The number of familiar
   _____
   should be increased.

8. The _____ level
   should be decreased.

9. Listening to _____
   may calm residents.

8. Identify what must be done if a restraint is ordered

Crossword Puzzle

Across

2. The medical term for skin that is blue-
   tinged, gray, or pale

3. Something that restraints cannot be used for

4. The minimum number of minutes at which
   a resident in a physical restraint must be
   checked

Down

1. At a minimum, the number of hours at
   which restraints must be released

2. Device that must be placed within a resident's reach when the resident is restrained

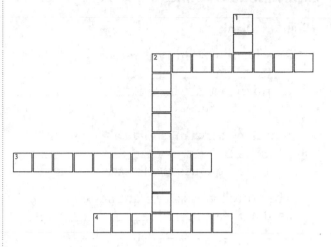

9. List safety guidelines for oxygen use

True or False

1. ____ A nursing assistant should adjust a
   resident's oxygen levels if the resident
   is having trouble breathing.

2. ____ Oxygen is a dangerous fire hazard.

3. ____ Smoking should not be allowed any-
   where around oxygen equipment.

4. ____ Fire hazards that should be removed
   from residents' rooms include electric
   razors and hair dryers.

5. ____ Combustion means that something is
   full and ready to burst.

6. ____ The use of lighters is allowed around
   oxygen.

7. ____ Alcohol and nail polish remover are
   considered flammable liquids.

8. ____ Oxygen tubing should remain lying
   flat underneath the resident at all
   times.

9. ____ Vaseline can be used to soften the
   skin for a resident who has irritation
   from the nasal cannula.

10. Identify safety guidelines for intravenous (IV) lines

Fill in the Blank

1. A resident with an IV is receiving

   _____,
   nutrition, or _____
   through a vein.

2. A nursing assistant should always wear

   _____
   if she has to touch the IV area.

3. The arm that has an IV line should not be used to measure _____

   _____.

4. The NA should not disconnect the IV line from the _____ or turn off the

   _____.

5. If the needle or

   _____ has fallen
   out or moves out of the vein, the NA should report to the nurse.

6. An _____

   is the administration of fluids into surrounding tissue.

7. The NA should report to the nurse if the resident complains of

   _____
   or has difficulty _____.

11. Discuss fire safety and explain the RACE and PASS acronyms

Multiple Choice

1. What are the three things needed for a fire to occur?
   (A) Heat, cold, matches
   (B) Heat, fuel, oxygen
   (C) Heat, nitrogen, oxygen
   (D) Heat, electrical current, fuel

2. PASS is an acronym used to explain how to operate a fire extinguisher. The letters stand for
   (A) Pull the pin, Aim at the base of the fire, Squeeze the handle, Sweep back and forth at the base
   (B) Push the handle, Aim at the base of the fire, Spray the water, Sweep back and forth at the base
   (C) Push the extinguisher, Aim at the fire, Squeeze the handle, Spray in a circle
   (D) Pull the pin, Access the lock, Squeeze the handle, Spray from top of the fire down

3. If clothing catches fire, it is best for the person to
   (A) Jump up and down to fan the flames
   (B) Stay still and drop to the ground
   (C) Start running
   (D) Find a buddy to exit the area together

12. List general safety steps for working in a healthcare facility

True or False

1. ____ Living or working in a facility means a person is safe from all crime.

2. ____ Very few people go in and out of a facility during the day.

3. ____ It is best for a nursing assistant to watch for suspicious behavior and report it immediately.

4. ____ It is a smart idea for a nursing assistant to take valuables to work so that he can keep an eye on them.

5. ____ A nursing assistant should not leave a resident alone with a visitor or staff member who makes her uneasy.

6. ____ To promote safety, an NA should share her personal information with anyone who asks.

8

Emergency Care, First Aid, and Disasters

1. Review the key terms in Learning Objective 1 before completing the workbook exercises

2. Demonstrate how to respond to medical emergencies

Short Answer

1. When a nursing assistant is assessing an emergency situation, what should he do?

_____

_____

_____

_____

_____

_____

2. When a nursing assistant is assessing a victim in a medical emergency, what should he do?

_____

_____

_____

_____

_____

_____

_____

_____

_____

_____

_____

_____

_____

_____

_____

_____

_____

3. Demonstrate knowledge of first aid procedures

Crossword Puzzle

Across

2. Medical term for vomiting

4. Sudden stopping/cessation of the heartbeat

5. Medical term for fainting or temporary loss of consciousness

Down

1. Stopping/cessation of breathing

3. Way to help someone who is choking by placing both hands around a person's waist and pulling inward and upward

4. Abbreviation for medical procedures used when a person's heart and lungs have stopped working

Name: _____

True or False

1. _____ Normally when a person is choking, she lies face down on the ground.

2. _____ The nursing assistant should leave a choking victim alone in order to find someone to help her.

3. _____ Before giving abdominal thrusts, the nursing assistant should ask the victim if he is choking.

4. _____ A person in shock should sit upright until symptoms improve.

5. _____ After notifying the nurse, the first step a nursing assistant should take when trying to control bleeding is to put on gloves.

6. _____ When blood seeps through a pad that is being used to control bleeding, it should be removed and replaced with a clean pad.

7. _____ Applying butter to a serious burn will help reduce the chance of infection.

8. _____ If a person appears likely to faint and is sitting down, the nursing assistant should have her bend forward and put her head between her knees.

9. _____ The medical term for fainting is *epistaxis*.

10. _____ When a person has vomited, it is important to check vomitus for blood or medication.

11. _____ Men are more likely than women to deny that they are having a heart attack.

12. _____ If a nursing assistant suspects a person is having a heart attack, she should give him water right away.

13. _____ The medical term for a heart attack is *transient ischemic attack*.

14. _____ Insulin reaction results from too much insulin or too little food.

15. _____ Diabetic ketoacidosis may be caused by undiagnosed diabetes.

16. _____ If a resident is having a seizure, the nursing assistant should put his fingers inside the resident's mouth to clear any food.

17. _____ The response time to a suspected stroke is important, as early treatment can reduce the severity of the stroke.

18. _____ Slurred speech and facial droop are two important signs to report that may signal a stroke is beginning.

Matching

For each medical emergency listed below, write the letter of the correct sign or symptom or response. Use each letter only once.

1. _____ Bleeding

2. _____ Burn

3. _____ Choking

4. _____ Diabetic ketoacidosis

5. _____ Fainting (syncope)

6. _____ Insulin reaction (hypoglycemia)

7. _____ Myocardial infarction

8. _____ Nosebleed (epistaxis)

9. _____ Poisoning

10. _____ Seizure

11. ____ Shock

12. ____ Stroke

13. ____ Vomiting (emesis)

(A) Signs of this include pale or cyanotic skin, staring, increased pulse and respiration rates, low blood pressure, and extreme thirst.

(B) The NA should hold a thick sterile pad directly against the wound.

(C) Signs of this include severe pain in the chest, anxiety, and heartburn or indigestion.

(D) Performing abdominal thrusts may help with this emergency.

(E) The NA should apply firm pressure on both sides of the nose, up near the bridge, if this occurs.

(F) Ointment, salve, or grease should not be used as treatment.

(G) If a person is sitting, the NA can have her bend forward and place her head between her knees if she is able.

(H) Signs of this include use of inappropriate words, loss of bowel and bladder control, and arm numbness.

(I) When this occurs, the NA should not try to stop it or restrain the person.

(J) Sweet or fruity breath is a symptom.

(K) If this occurs, it is a good idea to give the person a glass of fruit juice or milk immediately.

(L) Providing mouth care after this happens is helpful.

(M) Signs of this include vomiting and heavy, difficult breathing.

4. Explain the nursing assistant's role on a code team

Fill in the Blank

1. Facilities use codes to inform staff of

   _____

   without alarming residents and visitors.

2. *Code Red* usually means

   _____,

   and *Code Blue* usually means

   _____.

3. The _____
   is the team chosen for a shift to respond in case of a resident emergency.

4. Staff on the code team may be asked to get a special _____
   or other emergency equipment.

5. Nursing assistants may be asked to perform

   _____

   during CPR.

5. Describe guidelines for responding to disasters

Short Answer

1. What kinds of disasters are most likely to occur in your area?

   _____

   _____

   _____

   _____

   _____

   _____

   _____

   _____

2. Describe the way nursing assistants should respond to disasters.

   _____

   _____

   _____

   _____

   _____

   _____

   _____

   _____

9

Admission, Transfer, Discharge, and Physical Exams

1. Review the key terms in Learning Objective 1 before completing the workbook exercises

2. List factors for families choosing a facility

Short Answer

1. What are three sources of information that families may use to guide them in choosing a facility for a loved one?

_____

_____

_____

_____

_____

2. Why do you think family members ask questions before deciding on a facility for their loved one?

_____

_____

_____

_____

_____

_____

_____

3. Explain the nursing assistant's role in the emotional adjustment of a new resident

Scenario
Read the following scenario and answer the questions that follow.

A new resident is having a hard time. She mostly cries in her room and refuses to participate in any activity. A nursing assistant stops by her room to measure her blood pressure. When he sees her crying by the window, he sighs loudly and rolls his eyes. "You're lucky I'm here," he says. "Nobody else knows how to deal with emotional residents."

He continues, "In fact, last week the resident in room 102 couldn't stop crying when he found out he has colon cancer. I was the only one he would talk to."

The resident continues to cry softly while the NA measures her blood pressure. "I don't know why you're so sad," he says. "I'd be happy if I could be somewhere where I got all my meals cooked and my room cleaned. Plus, there's lots of other old folks here to talk to."

He leaves her room and realizes he forgot to note the resident's blood pressure. Not wanting to deal with her again, he thinks for a moment and writes down some numbers.

1. Name seven things the NA could have done to take better care of the new resident.

_____

_____

_____

Name: _____

_____
_____
_____
_____
_____
_____
_____
_____
_____
_____
_____

2. List five reasons why moving into a care facility is a big emotional adjustment for new residents.

_____
_____
_____
_____
_____
_____
_____
_____
_____

4. Describe the nursing assistant's role in the admission process

True or False

1. ____ In order to keep a new resident occupied, the nursing assistant should let him figure out how to use the bed controls and the call light.

2. ____ A new resident's admission pack may include soap, a bedpan, and a water pitcher and cup.

3. ____ It is better for the nursing assistant to wait until the resident has already arrived to start preparing her room.

4. ____ The resident should not feel as if he is an inconvenience; he should feel welcome and wanted.

5. ____ It is important for the nursing assistant to introduce new residents to other residents and staff members.

6. ____ Baseline measurements are taken approximately six months after a resident is admitted to a care facility.

7. ____ A change in a resident's weight does not need to be reported as long as the gain or loss is within five pounds.

8. ____ Residents who cannot get out of bed cannot have their height or weight measured.

9. ____ When measuring height, the nursing assistant should remember that there are eight inches in a foot.

10. ____ One kilogram equals 2.2 pounds.

5. Explain the nursing assistant's role during an in-house transfer of a resident

Fill in the Blank

1. _____ is always hard. This may be especially true if the resident is _____ or his condition has _____.

2. Nursing assistants should try to make the transfer as _____ as possible for residents.

3. The nursing assistant should _____ the resident's personal items carefully to avoid damaging or losing them.

4. After the resident is in her new room, the nursing assistant should _____ her to everyone.

5. When leaving the resident's room, the nursing assistant should report to the

_____

in charge of the resident.

6. Explain the nursing assistant's role in the discharge of a resident

Multiple Choice

1. When does a resident's discharge from the facility become official?
   (A) After the doctor writes the discharge order that releases the resident to leave the facility
   (B) After the resident is informed of the discharge
   (C) After the resident leaves the facility
   (D) When the nurse gives the resident instructions to be followed after discharge

2. Which of the following is the nursing assistant's responsibility during discharge?
   (A) Collecting and packing the resident's belongings
   (B) Giving the resident any special dietary instructions
   (C) Writing the discharge order
   (D) Reviewing medications that the resident needs to take

3. A nursing assistant is responsible for the resident until
   (A) The discharge order has been written by the doctor
   (B) The resident's items are packed, and the inventory list has been checked
   (C) The resident is outside the facility
   (D) The resident is safely in the vehicle with the doors closed

7. Describe the nursing assistant's role during physical exams

Multiple Choice

1. What are the nursing assistant's duties during residents' physical exams?
   (A) Performing the exams
   (B) Giving injections
   (C) Diagnosing illness or disease
   (D) Gathering equipment for the doctor or nurse

2. In which position is the resident placed for examination of the breasts, chest, abdomen, and perineal area?
   (A) Dorsal recumbent position
   (B) Lithotomy position
   (C) Knee-chest position
   (D) Trendelenburg position

3. Which of the following pieces of equipment is used to measure blood pressure?
   (A) Reflex hammer
   (B) Thermometer
   (C) Sphygmomanometer
   (D) Otoscope

4. In which position is the resident in stirrups in order to examine the vagina?
   (A) Sims' position
   (B) Lithotomy position
   (C) Knee-chest position
   (D) Prone position

5. Which position is used to examine the rectum or the vagina?
   (A) Lateral position
   (B) Lithotomy position
   (C) Knee-chest position
   (D) Prone position

10

Bedmaking and Unit Care

1. Review the key terms in Learning Objective 1 before completing the workbook exercises

2. Discuss the importance of sleep

Fill in the Blank

1. _____ is a natural period of rest for the mind and body during which _____ is restored.

2. Sleep is needed to replace old _____ with new ones and provide new energy to _____.

3. _____ are natural rhythms or cycles related to body functions.

4. The _____ is the 24-hour day-night cycle.

3. Describe types of sleep disorders

Matching
Use each letter only once.

1. ____ Bruxism

2. ____ Insomnia

3. ____ Parasomnias

4. ____ REM behavior disorder

5. ____ Sleep apnea

6. ____ Sleep talking

7. ____ Somnambulism

(A) Talking during sleep

(B) Grinding and clenching the teeth

(C) Sleepwalking

(D) Inability to fall asleep or to remain asleep

(E) Sleep disorders

(F) Talking, often along with violent movements, during REM sleep

(G) Disruption of breathing while sleeping

4. Identify factors affecting sleep

Scenario
Read the following scenario and answer the questions that follow.

New resident Anne Ross has been having trouble sleeping. She generally has dinner, dessert, and coffee around 8:30 p.m. every day. Her husband recently died in the home they shared for 24 years. After his death, she started a new medication to help with her depression. Her roommate Riva likes to sleep with the light on because she frequently has to use the bathroom. Sometimes Riva is unable to make it to the bathroom in time and has to call a nursing assistant for help. The nursing assistant will change the sheets and help Riva clean herself as quickly as possible.

1. List five factors that could be affecting Anne's ability to sleep.

_____

_____

_____

_____

Name: _____

_____

_____

_____

_____

_____

_____

2. For each factor you listed above, suggest a solution that might help Anne sleep better.

_____

_____

_____

_____

_____

_____

_____

_____

_____

_____

_____

_____

_____

_____

_____

_____

3. List four problems that can be caused by not sleeping well.

_____

_____

_____

_____

_____

_____

_____

5. Describe a standard resident unit and equipment

Short Answer

For each of the following, make a check mark (✓) beside the standard equipment found in most resident units.

1. _____ Overbed table

2. _____ Mechanical lift

3. _____ Call light

4. _____ Bible

5. _____ Bed

6. _____ Bedpan

7. _____ Massage table

8. _____ Emesis basin

True or False

1. _____ A nursing assistant must always knock and wait for permission before entering a resident's room.

2. _____ Residents' personal items are not very important to them.

3. _____ If a nursing assistant notices a safety hazard in a resident's room, she should remove it immediately.

4. _____ Personal articles can be stored in the bedside stand.

5. _____ Bedpans should be stored on overbed tables when not being used.

6. _____ When making a bed, the nursing assistant should place the soiled linen on the overbed table.

6. Explain how to clean a resident unit and equipment

Multiple Choice

1. General care of the resident's unit must be done
   (A) Once a day
   (B) Whenever needed throughout the day
   (C) Once a week
   (D) Only when the resident requests that it be done

2. Which of the following is an example of disposable equipment?
    (A) Bedpan
    (B) Stethoscope
    (C) Gloves
    (D) Blood pressure cuff

3. The call light must always be kept
    (A) Within the resident's reach
    (B) Near the door
    (C) On the bedside stand
    (D) On the overbed table

4. After a resident is transferred, discharged, or dies, which of the following tasks should be completed by the nursing assistant?
    (A) Notifying people on the facility's waiting list that a room is ready
    (B) Removing equipment and supplies
    (C) Discarding the resident's remaining personal items
    (D) Repairing damaged or broken furniture

7. Discuss types of beds and demonstrate proper bedmaking

Multiple Choice

1. Using proper body mechanics when making a bed means that the nursing assistant should
    (A) Keep her knees locked and close together
    (B) Lower the bed to the lowest possible position
    (C) Bend her knees
    (D) Raise the bed so that it is positioned at the NA's head level

2. Which of the following is true of dirty linen?
    (A) It should be shaken to remove airborne contaminants before being placed in a hamper.
    (B) It should be rolled so that the dirty side is facing inward.
    (C) It should be rolled so that the dirty side is facing outward.
    (D) It should be placed on the floor after being removed from the bed.

3. Which of the following is a type of bed that is made while the resident is in the bed?
    (A) An unoccupied bed
    (B) An occupied bed
    (C) An open bed
    (D) A surgical bed

4. Where should the nursing assistant place clean linen when making a resident's bed?
    (A) On a clean surface within reach, such as an overbed table
    (B) On top of the hamper
    (C) On top of the counter in the resident's bathroom
    (D) On a clean towel on the floor

5. The branch of medicine that deals with the causes, prevention, and treatment of obesity is called
    (A) Obstetrics
    (B) Bariatrics
    (C) Oncology
    (D) Gastroenterology

6. An alternating pressure mattress is designed to
    (A) Sound an alarm when the resident gets out of bed
    (B) Be firmer under the resident's head and torso, but softer under his legs and feet
    (C) Alternate pressure to ensure one area of the body does not rest on a certain spot for too long
    (D) Control a resident's sleep-wake cycle with varying pressure settings

7. Which of the following is true about bariatric beds?
    (A) Bariatric beds are rated for residents up to 250 lbs.
    (B) Bariatric beds are higher than standard beds.
    (C) Bariatric beds have no upper weight limit.
    (D) Bariatric beds are closer to the floor than standard beds.

8. In which position should the resident's bed remain while the resident is in it?
   (A) Raised head and foot of the bed
   (B) Lowest
   (C) Highest
   (D) Directly on the floor

9. How should clean linen be carried?
   (A) Clean linen should be carried away from the NA's uniform.
   (B) Clean linen should be carried in a protective bag or case.
   (C) Clean linen should be carried against a resident's body.
   (D) Clean linen should be carried only by a member of the custodial department.

10. In which of the following scenarios should the NA immediately change a resident's linens?
    (A) The resident has eaten a meal in bed.
    (B) The resident has had an episode of incontinence.
    (C) The resident has taken a day trip and will be gone for several hours.
    (D) The resident has complained that the room is too cool.

11. What is the difference between a closed bed and an open bed?
    (A) A closed bed has the bedspread, blankets, and pillows in place, while an open bed has the linen folded down to the foot of the bed.
    (B) A closed bed will have top linen fanfolded along one edge, while an open bed has the bedspread pulled up to the top of the bed.
    (C) A closed bed does not have a bottom sheet in place, while an open bed does.
    (D) A closed bed has straps to secure the resident while in bed, while an open bed does not.

11

Positioning, Moving, and Lifting

1. Review the key terms in Learning Objective 1 before completing the workbook exercises

2. Explain body alignment and review the principles of body mechanics

Fill in the Blank

1. The nursing assistant should

   _____
   the load.

2. The nursing assistant should think ahead,

   _____,
   and communicate the move.

3. The nursing assistant should check her base
   of _____
   and be sure she has firm

   _____.

4. The nursing assistant should

   _____
   what she is lifting.

5. The nursing assistant should keep her back

   _____.

6. The nursing assistant should begin in a
   squatting position and lift with her

   _____.

7. The nursing assistant should

   _____
   her stomach muscles when beginning the
   lift.

8. The nursing assistant should keep the object

   _____
   to her body.

9. The nursing assistant should

   _____

   when possible rather than lifting.

3. Explain why position changes are important for bedbound residents and describe basic body positions

Matching
Use each letter only once.

1. ____ Dangling

2. ____ Draw sheet

3. ____ Fowler's

4. ____ Lateral

5. ____ Logrolling

6. ____ Positioning

7. ____ Prone

8. ____ Shearing

9. ____ Sims'

10. ____ Supine

(A) Semi-sitting body position (45 to 60 degrees)

(B) An extra sheet placed on top of the bottom
    sheet to help prevent skin damage caused by
    shearing

(C) Helping residents into positions that pro-
    mote comfort and health

(D) Body position in which the resident is lying
    on his abdomen

(E) Sitting up with the legs hanging over the
    side of the bed in order to regain balance

(F) Body position in which a resident is lying on either side

(G) Left side-lying body position in which the upper knee is flexed and raised toward the chest

(H) Body position in which the resident is lying flat on his back

(I) Rubbing or friction resulting from the skin moving one way and the bone underneath it remaining fixed or moving in the opposite direction

(J) Method of turning a resident as a unit, without disturbing the alignment of the body

Short Answer

1. At a minimum, how often should bedbound residents be repositioned? How often should residents in wheelchairs be repositioned?

_____
_____
_____
_____
_____

2. List three things that a nursing assistant should check a resident's skin for each time a resident is repositioned.

_____
_____
_____
_____
_____
_____
_____
_____

4. Describe how to safely transfer residents

Multiple Choice

1. How should a nursing assistant transfer a resident who has a stronger side and a weaker side?
   (A) The weaker side moves first.
   (B) The stronger side moves first.
   (C) Both sides must move together at the same time.
   (D) The left side moves first.

2. The science of designing equipment, areas, and tasks to make them safer and to suit the worker's abilities is called
   (A) Musculoskeletal motion
   (B) Robotics
   (C) Ergonomics
   (D) Body mechanics

3. Which of the following is a proper guideline for resident transfers?
   (A) Whenever the nursing assistant can, she should manually lift the resident from one place to another.
   (B) Having a zero-lift policy in place means that a nursing assistant should be able to lift the resident on her own, without help.
   (C) Safety is a lesser concern while transferring a resident than it is while positioning a resident.
   (D) It is important for the nursing assistant to get the help she needs when lifting a resident.

4. Which of the following is true of transfer belts?
   (A) They are called slide belts when used to help residents walk.
   (B) They are used most often for residents with fragile bones or recent fractures.
   (C) They fit around the resident's waist, over his clothes.
   (D) They are the same as mechanical lifts.

5. Slide boards are used for
   (A) Transferring residents who cannot bear weight on their legs from one sitting position to another
   (B) Helping weak residents ambulate for longer distances
   (C) Easier lifting of residents who can only bear weight on one leg
   (D) Transferring weak residents who are standing to a sitting position

6. Which of the following is true of using a wheelchair?
   (A) A resident's hips should be positioned close to the front of the chair.
   (B) When moving down a ramp, the NA should go down forward, with the resident facing the bottom of the ramp.
   (C) When using an elevator, the NA should turn the chair around so that the resident faces forward.
   (D) The wheels of the wheelchair should be unlocked before the NA transfers a resident out of the wheelchair.

7. Which of the following is true of mechanical lifts?
   (A) Mechanical lifts help protect staff and residents from injury during lifting.
   (B) Mechanical lifts are commonly used to transfer residents into ambulances.
   (C) Mechanical lifts are often used in place of wheelchairs as a way for residents to move around the facility.
   (D) Mechanical lifts are used in the dining room to help with safe food service.

8. For a resident to be able to use a toilet, he must be able to
   (A) Walk to the toilet without assistance
   (B) Stand up without assistance
   (C) Bear some weight on his legs
   (D) Transfer himself from a wheelchair to the toilet without assistance

5. Discuss ambulation

Multiple Choice

1. Ambulation is another term for
   (A) Logrolling or turning
   (B) Riding or rolling
   (C) Dangling or sitting
   (D) Walking or moving

2. Before assisting a resident to ambulate, her feet should be
   (A) Flat on the floor
   (B) Pointed to the side
   (C) Pointed upward
   (D) Barefoot

3. When helping a resident with a visual impairment walk, the nursing assistant should
   (A) Pull the gait belt to help the resident walk
   (B) Walk slightly behind the resident
   (C) Walk slightly in front of the resident
   (D) Stay about 12 inches away from the resident's side

Positioning, Moving, and Lifting

12
Personal Care

1. Review the key terms in Learning Objective 1 before completing the workbook exercises

2. Explain personal care of residents

True or False

1. _____ Regular grooming helps keep a person clean and healthy.

2. _____ All residents will be bathed in the morning after they wake up.

3. _____ The nursing assistant should insist that residents brush their teeth before eating breakfast.

4. _____ *Grooming* is the term to describe practices to keep the body clean, while *hygiene* includes practices like fingernail, foot, and hair care.

5. _____ Helping residents with their activities of daily living (ADLs) is outside of a nursing assistant's scope of practice.

6. _____ The nursing assistant should perform as much personal care as possible for the resident so that the resident does not become frustrated.

7. _____ Residents may be embarrassed by having someone else provide personal care.

8. _____ Residents have the right to choose what they want to wear, including jewelry.

9. _____ Residents should be left alone during bathing to promote independence.

10. _____ The nursing assistant should let the resident know that he is allowed to use the toilet for only a few minutes.

11. _____ The nursing assistant should keep residents covered as much as possible when bathing and dressing them.

3. Describe different types of baths and list observations to make about the skin during bathing

Short Answer

1. List the four basic types of baths. For each one, list one type of resident for which this bath is best suited.

_____

_____

_____

_____

_____

_____

_____

_____

_____

_____

_____

Name: _____

2. How is the decision made about which kind of bath a resident will receive?

_____
_____
_____
_____
_____
_____

3. List ten things to observe and report during personal care and bathing.

_____
_____
_____
_____
_____
_____
_____
_____
_____
_____
_____
_____

4. Explain safety guidelines for bathing

Short Answer

Place a check mark (✓) next to the ways to promote safety during bathing.

1. ____ Maintaining a water temperature of 115 degrees Fahrenheit

2. ____ Using scented bath oils

3. ____ Using grab bars

4. ____ Keeping the bathing supplies within reach

5. ____ Leaving the resident alone

6. ____ Keeping the floor dry

7. ____ Using talcum powder

8. ____ Using nonslip mats

5. List the order in which body parts are washed during bathing

Short Answer

1. Why is it important to follow a specific order when bathing a person?

_____
_____
_____
_____
_____
_____

2. State the general rule for the order of washing body parts during bathing.

_____
_____
_____
_____
_____

Labeling

Look at the figure below. In the blanks provided, number the parts of the body in the order in which they should be bathed.

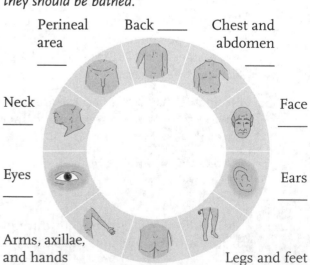

Perineal area ____   Back ____   Chest and abdomen ____

Neck ____   Face ____

Eyes ____   Ears ____

Arms, axillae, and hands ____   Buttocks ____   Legs and feet ____

6. Explain how to assist with bathing

Multiple Choice

1. What opportunity does bathing a resident give the nursing assistant?
   (A) It allows the nursing assistant to talk to other nursing assistants.
   (B) It allows the nursing assistant to see if the resident needs to change her medications.
   (C) It allows the nursing assistant to observe the skin and report changes.
   (D) It allows the nursing assistant to understand how the resident feels about hygiene.

2. Which one of the following parts of the body should be washed every day?
   (A) Hair
   (B) Thighs
   (C) Back
   (D) Perineal area

3. When is a partial bath performed?
   (A) Every day
   (B) Only for testing purposes
   (C) On days when a complete bed bath, tub bath, or shower is not done
   (D) When a resident cannot get out of bed

4. To shampoo hair for a resident on a stretcher, the nursing assistant should
   (A) Transfer the resident to a bed
   (B) Transfer the resident to a chair in front of the sink
   (C) Bring the stretcher to the sink and adjust the height of the stretcher
   (D) Place a cup and a bucket full of warm water near the stretcher

5. What kind of equipment is used to help a resident into a whirlpool bath?
   (A) Gait belt
   (B) Slide board
   (C) Chair lift
   (D) Wheelchair

6. When performing perineal care, what is important to remember?
   (A) Washing from back to front
   (B) Using a lot of soap
   (C) Using a clean area of the cloth for each stroke
   (D) Cleaning the anal area before cleaning the perineal area

7. Describe how to perform a back rub

True or False

1. ____ It is inappropriate for a nursing assistant to give a resident a back rub.

2. ____ Back rubs help relax muscles and improve circulation.

3. ____ Back rubs need to be given to all residents.

4. ____ The position that is most comfortable for elderly people is lying on their stomachs (prone).

5. ____ Red areas over bony parts of the body should be massaged using long, smooth strokes.

8. Explain guidelines for performing mouth care

Matching
Use each letter only once.

1. ____ Edentulous

2. ____ Gingivitis

3. ____ Halitosis

4. ____ Plaque

5. ____ Tartar

(A) Inflammation of the gums

(B) Substance that accumulates on the teeth from food and bacteria

(C) Bad breath

(D) Hard deposits on teeth that are filled with bacteria and may cause gum disease and loose teeth

(E) Lacking teeth

Short Answer

1. List seven signs and symptoms to report during mouth care.

_____

_____

_____

_____

_____

_____

_____

_____

_____

_____

2. List five ways that a nursing assistant will assist a resident who can brush his own teeth.

_____

_____

_____

_____

_____

_____

_____

_____

_____

_____

9. Define *dentures* and explain care guidelines

Crossword Puzzle

Across

2. Must be worn by the nursing assistant when cleaning dentures

3. Dentures that are left uncovered can warp, dry out, or do this

4. A labeled one of these may be used to store dentures

5. A type of dental appliance that replaces missing or pulled teeth

6. Temperature of water that can warp dentures

7. When a person's dentures break, he can no longer do this

Down

1. Water temperature for denture storage so that they do not dry out and warp

4. Another word for artificial teeth

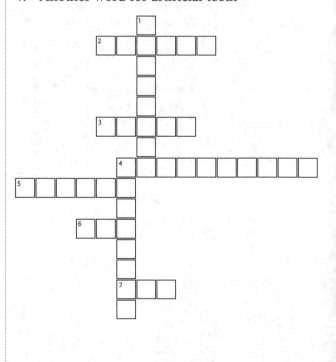

10. Discuss guidelines for performing mouth care for an unconscious resident

Multiple Choice

1. Why does mouth care need to be done frequently for residents who are unconscious?
   (A) Too much moisture collects in the mouth and needs to be removed
   (B) To encourage the growth of "good" bacteria in the mouth
   (C) The mouth becomes dry due to a lack of fluids, breathing through the mouth, and oxygen therapy
   (D) To help make it easier to chew food

2. Aspiration is
   (A) A crust that appears on the lips, gums, and teeth of people who are unconscious
   (B) A cause of unconsciousness
   (C) Inhalation of food, fluid, or foreign material into the lungs
   (D) A procedure used to create an artificial airway

3. One way to prevent aspiration is to
   (A) Turn unconscious residents on their backs before beginning mouth care
   (B) Avoid performing mouth care on unconscious residents
   (C) Use as little liquid as possible during mouth care
   (D) Use swabs soaked in large amounts of fluid to clean the mouth

4. Residents who are unconscious may still be able to
   (A) Hear
   (B) Dress themselves
   (C) Ambulate
   (D) Feed themselves

5. Which of the following statements is true of performing eye care for an unconscious resident?
   (A) The nursing assistant should use gloves when bathing the eye.
   (B) The nursing assistant should wipe from the outer area to the inner area of the eye when cleaning.
   (C) The nursing assistant should use the same washcloth to clean both eyes.
   (D) The nursing assistant should not speak to an unconscious resident while performing care.

11. Explain how to assist with grooming

True or False

1. ____ Appearance has very little to do with how people feel about themselves.

2. ____ The nursing assistant will make all the decisions about how to groom a resident.

3. ____ A nursing assistant must always wear gloves when shaving residents.

4. ____ All residents need to be shaved.

5. ____ Disposable shaving products should be discarded in the biohazard container for sharps.

6. ____ A safety razor is the safest and easiest razor to use.

7. ____ Fingernails can collect and harbor microorganisms.

8. ____ All facilities allow nursing assistants to clip residents' toenails regularly.

9. ____ A nursing assistant should trim a resident's hair when it is too long or if it becomes matted.

10. ____ Hair typically thins as a person ages.

11. ____ A nursing assistant should style a resident's hair like a little kid's hair is styled; for example, she should put it in two high ponytails.

12. _____   Lice do not typically spread very quickly.

13. _____   Most residents who have roommates will share their combs and brushes with each other.

14. _____   If a resident has one side of the body that is weaker than the other, the nursing assistant should refer to that side as the *involved* side.

15. _____   When dressing a resident who has a weaker side of the body, the nursing assistant should always begin with the stronger side.

16. _____   To promote comfort and better sleep, residents should wear pajamas all day long.

17. _____   Bras that fasten in the back are easier for female residents to manage by themselves.

18. _____   When helping a resident undress, the nursing assistant should begin with the stronger side.

13
Vital Signs

1. Review the key terms in Learning Objective 1 before completing the workbook exercises

2. Discuss the relationship of vital signs to health and well-being

Matching
Match each vital sign with the correct range.

1. _____ Axillary temperature

2. _____ Stage 1 hypertension

3. _____ Low blood pressure/hypotension

4. _____ Normal blood pressure

5. _____ Oral temperature

6. _____ Elevated blood pressure

7. _____ Normal pulse rate

8. _____ Rectal temperature

9. _____ Normal respiratory rate

10. _____ Temporal artery temperature

(A) 97.2°F–100.1°F

(B) 90–119 mm Hg and 60–79 mm Hg

(C) 97.6°F–99.6°F

(D) 120–129 mm Hg and less than 80 mm Hg

(E) 130–139 mm Hg or 80–89 mm Hg

(F) 60–100 per minute

(G) 12–20 per minute

(H) 98.6°F–100.6°F

(I) 96.6°F–98.6°F

(J) Below 90 mm Hg or below 60 mm Hg

Short Answer

1. Why is it important for a nursing assistant to report changes in vital signs to the nurse?

_____

_____

_____

_____

_____

_____

_____

_____

3. Identify factors that affect body temperature

Multiple Choice

1. Which of the following is the average temperature of the body?
   (A) 98.6°F
   (B) 96.6°F
   (C) 94.8°F
   (D) 99.6°F

2. The medical term for severe subnormal body temperature is
   (A) Dyspnea
   (B) Tachycardia
   (C) Hypothermia
   (D) Orthopnea

Vital Signs

3. How does a person's age affect body temperature?
   (A) An older person has lost protective fatty tissue, which may cause him to feel colder.
   (B) Skin thickens as a person ages, causing him to feel warmer.
   (C) An older person no longer exercises, which makes him feel colder.
   (D) An older person is ill most of the time, which means he feels hotter.

4. List guidelines for measuring body temperature

Short Answer
Mark an X by each person for whom an oral temperature should NOT be taken.

1. _____ Person is disoriented.

2. _____ Person has sores in his mouth.

3. _____ Person is 40 years old.

4. _____ Person is unconscious.

5. _____ Person has a broken leg.

6. _____ Person is likely to have a seizure.

7. _____ Person has a nasogastric tube.

8. _____ Person has had children.

Short Answer
For each statement below, write an O if it refers to oral temperature, an R for rectal temperature, a T for tympanic temperature, an A for axillary temperature, or TA for temporal artery temperature.

1. _____ Thermometer is usually color-coded red

2. _____ Thermometer is lubricated

3. _____ Noninvasive method of measuring temperature

4. _____ May be necessary for unconscious residents

5. _____ Thermometer is inserted only ¼ to ½ inch

6. _____ Site for taking temperature is the armpit

7. _____ Considered to be most accurate

8. _____ Earwax may cause an inaccurate reading

9. _____ Thermometer is inserted no more than one inch

10. _____ Thermometer is usually color-coded green or blue

11. _____ Probe is moved straight across the forehead

12. _____ Site for taking temperature is the ear

13. _____ Ear injury is possible

Short Answer
For each illustration of mercury-free thermometers shown below, write the temperature reading to the nearest tenth degree in the blanks provided.

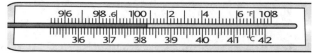

1. _____

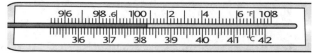

2. _____

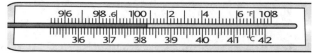

3. _____

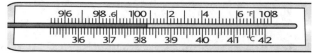

4. _____

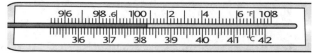

5. _____

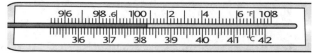

6. _____

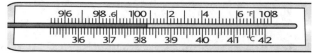

7. _____

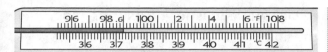

8. _____

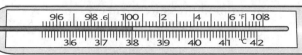

9. _____

10. _____

5. Explain pulse and respirations

Matching
Use each letter only once.

1. _____ Apnea

2. _____ BPM

3. _____ Bradycardia

4. _____ Cheyne-Stokes respiration

5. _____ Dilate

6. _____ Dyspnea

7. _____ Eupnea

8. _____ Expiration

9. _____ Inspiration

10. _____ Orthopnea

11. _____ Respiration

12. _____ Tachycardia

13. _____ Tachypnea

14. _____ Kussmaul breathing

(A) The absence of breathing

(B) To widen

(C) The process of inhaling air into the lungs and exhaling air out of the lungs

(D) Difficulty breathing

(E) Inhaling air into the lungs

(F) Slow heart rate—under 60 beats per minute

(G) Medical abbreviation for beats per minute

(H) Exhaling air out of the lungs

(I) Shortness of breath when lying down that is relieved by sitting up

(J) Alternating periods of slow, irregular respirations and rapid, shallow respirations, possibly along with periods of apnea

(K) Rapid heart rate—over 100 beats per minute

(L) Normal respirations

(M) Very deep, rapid breathing that is associated with diabetic ketoacidosis

(N) Rapid respirations—over 20 breaths per minute

6. List guidelines for counting pulse and respirations

Multiple Choice

1. The most common site for counting pulse beats is the
   (A) Apical pulse
   (B) Radial pulse
   (C) Brachial pulse
   (D) Femoral pulse

2. Respiration rate is counted directly after taking the pulse because
   (A) People tend to breathe more quickly if they know they are being observed
   (B) People tend to breathe more slowly if they know they are being observed
   (C) Breathing tends to be more regular if the person knows they are being observed
   (D) It saves time for the nursing assistant

3. Which of the following may be indicated if the radial pulse is less than the apical pulse?
   (A) Heart disease
   (B) Infection
   (C) Fever
   (D) Poor circulation to extremities

Vital Signs

7. Identify factors that affect blood pressure

Crossword Puzzle

Across

3. Regular amounts usually decrease a person's blood pressure

4. Medical term for low blood pressure

5. Top number in a blood pressure reading

Down

1. Medical term for high blood pressure

2. Bottom number in a blood pressure reading

6. Sudden drop in blood pressure when a person stands up

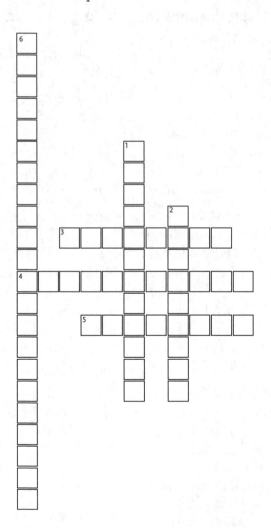

8. List guidelines for measuring blood pressure

True or False

1. _____ Blood pressure is measured with a device called a sphygmomanometer.

2. _____ As long as a stethoscope is used, the placement of the blood pressure cuff on the arm does not matter.

3. _____ An aneroid sphygmomanometer displays readings digitally.

4. _____ The apical pulse is the most commonly used pulse site to obtain a blood pressure reading.

5. _____ A blood pressure reading should not be measured on an arm that is being used for dialysis.

6. _____ Blood pressure readings may be taken while a resident is lying down, sitting up, and standing if he has orthostatic hypotension.

7. _____ A stethoscope is not required when measuring blood pressure electronically.

Short Answer

For each of the gauges shown below, record the blood pressure shown and answer the question.

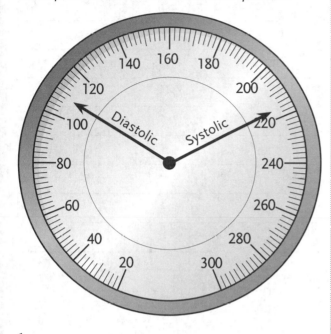

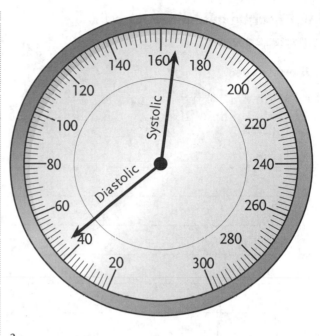

3. _____

   Is this reading within normal range?

   _____

1. _____

   Is this reading within normal range?

   _____

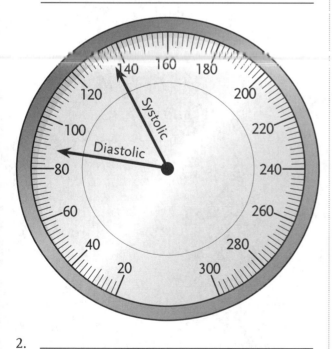

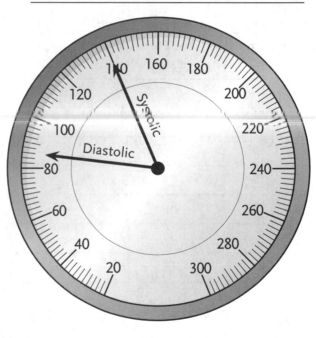

4. _____

   Is this reading within normal range?

   _____

2. _____

   Is this reading within normal range?

   _____

9. Describe guidelines for pain management

Short Answer

1. Have you ever been in pain for an extended period of time? If so, how did it affect your life?

    _____

    _____

    _____

    _____

    _____

    _____

    _____

2. List ten signs that a resident is in pain.

    _____

    _____

    _____

    _____

    _____

    _____

    _____

    _____

3. List five measures to reduce pain.

    _____

    _____

    _____

    _____

    _____

    _____

    _____

    _____

    _____

14

Nutrition and Fluid Balance

1. Review the key terms in Learning Objective 1 before completing the workbook exercises

2. Describe common nutritional problems of the elderly and the chronically ill

Crossword Puzzle

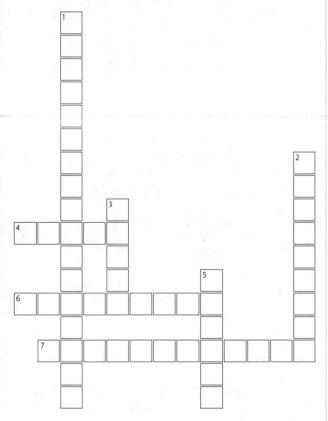

Across

4. One sense affected by aging and/or medication that affects the appetite

6. The medical term for difficulty swallowing

7. Lack of proper nutrition that results from insufficient food intake or an improper diet

Down

1. One disease that can make swallowing difficult

2. How the body uses food to maintain health

3. Problems with these make chewing difficult

5. When less of this is produced, eating and swallowing are affected

3. Describe cultural factors that influence food preferences

Short Answer

1. List three factors that influence food choices.

_____

_____

_____

_____

_____

2. Of the factors you listed above, which one has the most influence on your personal food choices and why?

_____

_____

_____

_____

_____

Name: _____

_____
_____
_____
_____
_____
_____
_____
_____
_____
_____

4. Identify six basic nutrients

Short Answer

Write the letter of the correct basic nutrient beside each description below. Use a W for water, F for fats, C for carbohydrates, P for proteins, V for vitamins, or M for minerals. Letters may be used more than once.

1. ____ Essential for tissue growth and repair

2. ____ A person can survive only a few days without this

3. ____ Monounsaturated and polyunsaturated are types

4. ____ The body does not make most of these nutrients; they can only be obtained through certain foods

5. ____ Give flavor to foods

6. ____ Add fiber to diets, which helps with solid waste elimination

7. ____ Help keep bones and teeth strong

8. ____ Help remove waste products from cells

9. ____ Can be fat-soluble or water-soluble

10. ____ Most essential nutrient for life

5. Explain the USDA's MyPlate

Short Answer

The USDA developed the MyPlate icon and website to help promote healthy eating practices. Looking at the MyPlate icon, fill in the food groups.

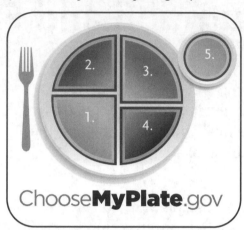

1. _____
2. _____
3. _____
4. _____
5. _____

Short Answer

Read each description and mark which food group it is describing—V for vegetables, F for fruits, G for grains, P for protein, and D for dairy. Multiple letters may be used for some descriptions.

1. ____ This group includes foods that retain their calcium content, such as yogurt and cheese.

2. ____ This includes all foods made from wheat, rice, oats, cornmeal, and barley.

3. ____ Plant sources of this include beans and vegetarian meat substitutes.

4. ____ Eating seafood twice a week in place of meat or poultry is recommended for this group.

5. ____ Most choices from this group should be fat-free or low-fat.

6. ____ This contains important sources of dietary fiber and many nutrients, including folic acid and vitamin C.

7. ____ Half of a person's plate should consist of choices from these two groups.

8. ____ At least half of all of these consumed should be "whole."

9. ____ One subgroup of these contains the bran, germ, and endosperm.

10. ____ These products contain calcium, potassium, vitamin D, and protein.

11. ____ Within this group, dark green, red, and orange types have the best nutritional content.

12. ____ Animal sources of this include meat, poultry, seafood, and eggs.

Short Answer

1. What is calorie balance?

_____

_____

_____

_____

_____

2. What are two things that contribute to overeating?

_____

_____

_____

3. List four types of foods that a person should eat more often.

_____

_____

_____

_____

_____

4. List three types of food that a person should eat less often.

_____

_____

_____

_____

5. List six types of food that are high in sodium.

_____

_____

_____

_____

_____

_____

_____

_____

_____

_____

_____

_____

6. What should be consumed instead of sugary drinks?

_____

_____

_____

6. Explain the role of the dietary department

Multiple Choice

1. Which of the following is a responsibility of the dietary department?
   (A) The department writes the medical order for which type of special diet each resident requires.
   (B) The department prepares food in such a way that residents are able to manage.
   (C) The department is responsible for making sure that residents are ready for their meals.
   (D) The department prepares food for residents' families.

2. Which of the following information is included on a resident's diet card?
    (A) Special diets, allergies, likes and dislikes, and other dietary instructions
    (B) Intake and output records
    (C) Amount of activity
    (D) Health department survey results

3. Which of the following is a guideline for how nursing assistants should read menus to residents and assist them with selecting their choices?
    (A) The NA should speak quickly and loudly.
    (B) The NA should not include beverage choices.
    (C) The NA should make selections sound appetizing.
    (D) The NA should encourage nutritious choices, but should make the final decision, even if the resident prefers something else.

7. Explain the importance of following diet orders and identify special diets

Short Answer
For each of the following, list the kind of special diet it is describing.

1. Resident is drinking fluids that a person can see through.

    _____

2. Resident has kidney or liver disease and is eating vegetables and starches and reducing protein intake.

    _____

3. Resident is eating whole grains and raw fruits and vegetables.

    _____

4. Resident is trying to lose weight.

    _____

5. Resident is making the transition from a liquid diet to a regular diet.

    _____

6. Resident has severe heart or kidney disease and has fluid intake monitored.

    _____

7. Resident has a serious burn that is healing and is eating lean meats, eggs, and protein shakes.

    _____

8. Resident is taking diuretics and eating bananas, oranges, and sweet potatoes and yams.

    _____

9. Resident has trouble chewing and swallowing and cannot tolerate a regular or soft mechanical diet.

    _____

10. Resident has heart disease and is limiting his salt intake.

    _____

11. Resident has a bowel disorder and is decreasing intake of grains, dairy, and coffee.

    _____

12. Resident is consuming clear liquids with the addition of cream soups, milk, and ice cream.

    _____

13. Resident's food is prepared with a blender or food processor.

    _____

14. Resident has intestinal problems and is avoiding spicy foods and citrus fruits.

    _____

15. Resident is trying to gain weight after surgery or an illness.

    _____

16. Resident is counting carbohydrates.

    _____

17. Resident has celiac disease, and foods containing wheat flour are eliminated from the diet.

    _____

18. Resident cannot digest the sugar found in milk and other products, but is allowed soy milk.

    _____

19. Resident does not eat meat for ethical reasons, but chooses to eat eggs and dairy products.

_____

20. Resident eats only plant-based foods.

_____

21. Resident eats foods that contain more of this mineral, such as spinach and kale, legumes, lean meats, and enriched cereals.

_____

8. Explain thickened liquids and identify three basic thickening consistencies

True or False

1. ____ Residents with dysphagia are evaluated to determine if they should consume thickened liquids.

2. ____ Thickened liquids move down the throat more slowly and limit the risk of choking.

3. ____ Residents who need to consume thickened liquids are still allowed to drink nonthickened coffee and water.

4. ____ The three types of thickened liquids generally used by facilities are nectar thick, honey thick, and pudding thick.

5. ____ Residents can drink liquids that are pudding thick from a cup with or without a straw.

9. List ways to identify and prevent unintended weight loss

Fill in the Blank

1. Unintended weight loss may be due to a(n) _____ condition or a(n) _____ diet.

2. Unintended weight loss puts a person at a greater risk for _____.

3. It is important for nursing assistants to _____ any weight loss they notice.

4. Staff may change special _____ orders due to weight loss.

5. Warning signs of unintended weight loss include the resident having _____ that do not fit properly or difficulty chewing or _____.

6. Signs that a resident is malnourished include a feeling of _____ throughout the body, weight loss, frequent _____, and problems with _____.

7. The nursing assistant should report any decrease in _____ to the nurse.

8. The nursing assistant should _____ food to the resident's preferences.

9. The nursing assistant should check _____ and meal trays to make sure residents are receiving the correct food.

10. The nursing assistant should talk about food being served in a _____ way to encourage eating.

10. Describe how to make dining enjoyable for residents

True or False

1. ____ Mealtimes are often the most anticipated times of the day for residents.

2. ____ Nursing assistants should encourage residents to eat as little as possible so that they do not gain too much weight.

3. ____ Staff should honor residents' requests to sit with friends.

4. ____ The best position for eating is reclining about 45 degrees.

5. ____ Dining tables should be adjusted to the right height for wheelchairs.

Name: _____

6. _____ Food should be served promptly to maintain correct temperature.

7. _____ Residents should be given assistive devices for eating if needed.

8. _____ If a resident needs his food cut for him before eating, this should be done at the dining table.

9. _____ Residents must eat whatever food is served, even if it is not what they want.

11. Describe how to serve meal trays and assist with eating

Multiple Choice

1. When serving meals to residents, a nursing assistant should
   (A) Check the diet card and identify the resident before serving the meal tray
   (B) Do as much as possible for each resident so that the meal can be finished more quickly
   (C) Leave the door of the food cart open so that the food is not too hot when served
   (D) Serve one resident at each table before going back to serve the second resident at each table

2. Which of the following is a way that a nursing assistant can promote residents' dignity during mealtime?
   (A) The nursing assistant should let residents know which food they need to eat first.
   (B) The nursing assistant should insist that residents wear bibs to keep their clothing free of food.
   (C) The nursing assistant should discourage conversation during mealtimes so that residents will be able to eat more quickly.
   (D) The nursing assistant should say positive things about the food being served.

3. Which of the following is a guideline that a nursing assistant should follow for helping residents during mealtimes?
   (A) The nursing assistant should mix all of the food on the plate together so that residents will be more likely to eat it.
   (B) The nursing assistant should tell residents which foods look appetizing and which do not.
   (C) The nursing assistant should blow on food that is too hot to get it to cool down more quickly.
   (D) The nursing assistant should respect residents' refusals to eat but report them to the nurse.

4. In which position should a resident be for eating?
   (A) Partially reclining
   (B) Sitting upright
   (C) Flat on his or her back
   (D) On his or her side with the head raised

12. Describe how to assist residents with special needs

Short Answer
For each of the following problems with eating, list one technique for helping a resident eat.

1. Resident has had a stroke and has a weaker side.

   _____
   _____
   _____

2. Resident has Parkinson's disease.

   _____
   _____
   _____

3. Resident has a visual impairment.

   _____
   _____
   _____

4. Resident eats too quickly.

_____

_____

_____

5. Resident bites down on utensils.

_____

_____

_____

6. Resident cannot or will not chew.

_____

_____

_____

7. Resident will not stop chewing.

_____

_____

_____

8. Resident holds food in his mouth.

_____

_____

_____

9. Resident pockets food in his cheek.

_____

_____

_____

10. Resident has poor lip closure.

_____

_____

_____

11. Resident has no teeth or is missing teeth.

_____

_____

12. Resident has dentures that do not fit properly.

_____

_____

_____

_____

13. Resident has a change in vision.

_____

_____

_____

14. Resident has a protruding tongue or tongue thrust.

_____

_____

_____

15. Resident will not open his mouth.

_____

_____

_____

16. Resident falls asleep while eating.

_____

_____

_____

17. Resident chokes when drinking.

_____

_____

_____

18. Resident forgets to eat.

_____

_____

_____

19. Resident drools excessively.

_____

_____

_____

20. Resident has poor sitting balance.

_____

_____

_____

21. Resident tends to lean to one side.

_____

_____

_____

22. Resident tends to fall forward.

_____

_____

_____

23. Resident has poor neck control.

_____

_____

_____

13. Discuss dysphagia and list guidelines for preventing aspiration

Multiple Choice

1. Which of the following is a cause of dysphagia?
   (A) Problems with dentures
   (B) Problems with casts
   (C) Problems with splints
   (D) Problems with warm applications

2. Which of the following is a sign of dysphagia?
   (A) Eating very rapidly
   (B) Healthy enjoyment of eating
   (C) Normal breathing
   (D) Coughing during or after meals

3. Guidelines for preventing aspiration include the following:
   (A) Placing residents in a reclining position for eating and drinking
   (B) Placing food in the paralyzed side of the mouth
   (C) Offering at least three bites of food before offering a liquid
   (D) Making sure food is swallowed after each bite

14. Describe intake and output (I&O)

Short Answer

1. Ms. Brown just ate some lentil soup from a six-ounce container. The NA measures the leftover soup, which is about 35 milliliters. How many milliliters of soup did Ms. Brown eat?

_____

2. Record this resident's total intake and output:

1 glass apple juice	140 mL
1 cup coffee	110 mL
1 cup soup	170 mL
Total intake:	_____

11:00 a.m.	
Urinate x 1	220 mL output measured
1:00 p.m.	
Urinate x 1	260 mL output measured
Total output:	_____

3. A resident drinks three 4-ounce glasses of water. How many milliliters is this?

_____

4. A resident's urine output measures 15 ounces. How many milliliters is this?

_____

5. How many milliliters are equal to one ounce?

_____

6. For dinner the resident has six ounces of soup, an eight-ounce glass of cranberry juice, and four ounces of ice cream. How many milliliters is this?

_____

7. For breakfast the resident has three ounces of orange juice, four ounces of coffee, and four ounces of milk. How many milliliters is this?

_____

8. A resident has a fluid restriction and is limited to 720 milliliters in an eight-hour time period. How many ounces is this?

_____

9. For lunch a resident is served eight ounces of coffee, eight ounces of water, and 10 ounces of soup. He drinks half of the water, half of the coffee, and eats all of the soup. How many milliliters is this?

_____

15. List ways to identify and prevent dehydration

Multiple Choice

1. When a resident is dehydrated, he may have
   (A) Light-colored urine
   (B) Cracked lips
   (C) Moist mucous membranes
   (D) Regular bowel elimination

Short Answer

1. What should a nursing assistant do every time she sees a resident to help prevent dehydration?

_____

_____

_____

_____

2. How could a water pitcher being too heavy for a resident to lift contribute to dehydration?

_____

_____

_____

_____

_____

16. List signs and symptoms of fluid overload and describe conditions that may require fluid restrictions

Fill in the Blank

1. Fluid overload occurs when more fluid _____ the body than is _____ from the body.

2. Fluid overload can occur when the heart, _____, or lungs are not working properly.

3. Symptoms of fluid overload include weight _____, difficulty _____, and _____ heart rate.

4. The nursing assistant should check for _____ of the ankles, feet, fingers, or hands.

5. A(n) _____ order means the person must limit the daily amount of fluids to a level set by the doctor.

6. Reasons for fluid restrictions include recent _____, illness, a special _____, or having a feeding _____.

Name: _____

15

The Gastrointestinal System

1. Review the key terms in Learning Objective 1 before completing the workbook exercises

2. Explain key terms related to the body

Matching
Use each letter only once.

1. _____ Anatomy

2. _____ Biology

3. _____ Body systems

4. _____ Cells

5. _____ Homeostasis

6. _____ Organ

7. _____ Pathophysiology

8. _____ Physiology

9. _____ Tissues

(A) A group of cells that performs similar tasks; connective and nervous are examples

(B) The study of all life forms

(C) A structural unit in the human body that performs a specific function; the heart is an example

(D) The study of body structure

(E) The study of the disorders that occur in the body

(F) The condition in which all of the body's systems are balanced and are working at their best

(G) The basic structural units of all organisms

(H) Groups of organs that perform specific functions in the human body

(I) The study of how body parts function

3. Explain the structure and function of the gastrointestinal system

Fill in the Blank

1. The gastrointestinal system is made up of two sections: the
   _____
   and the _____
   _____

2. The epiglottis blocks food from entering the
   _____.

3. Most food and fluids are absorbed in the
   _____.

4. Feces is eliminated from the body by
   _____ through
   the anus.

5. The large intestine helps regulate water balance by absorbing _____
   and _____ and
   eliminating solid waste products as feces.

6. The functions of the gastrointestinal system
   are _____ and
   _____ of food,
   absorption of nutrients, and
   _____ of waste
   products.

4. Discuss changes in the gastrointestinal system due to aging

True or False

1. _____ As a person ages, he may find it harder to taste foods.

2. _____ An older person may be constipated more often.

3. _____ Difficulty chewing and swallowing may occur as a person ages.

4. _____ An increase in the ability to absorb vitamins and minerals is a normal change of aging.

5. _____ As a person ages, she may have an increase of saliva and other digestive fluids.

5. List normal qualities of stool and identify signs and symptoms to report about stool

Multiple Choice

1. Solid waste products eliminated by the colon are called
   (A) Tarry
   (B) Feces
   (C) Peristalsis
   (D) Chyme

2. What should normal stool look like?
   (A) It should be brown and formed.
   (B) It should be brown and loose.
   (C) It should be brown and hard.
   (D) It should be brown and liquid.

3. Which of the following is true of bowel elimination?
   (A) There should not be any pain when passing stool.
   (B) All people have a bowel movement once per day.
   (C) Fecal incontinence is a normal part of aging.
   (D) It is normal for blood to be in a person's stool.

6. List factors affecting bowel elimination and describe how to promote normal bowel elimination

Multiple Choice

1. The best position for bowel elimination is
   (A) Lying flat on the back
   (B) Squatting and leaning forward
   (C) Lying on the abdomen
   (D) Reclining at approximately 45 degrees

2. Which of the following might be increased in a resident's diet if constipation is a problem?
   (A) Butter
   (B) Red meat
   (C) Whole grains
   (D) Eggs

3. How should a nursing assistant place a standard bedpan?
   (A) The wider end should be aligned with the resident's buttocks.
   (B) The wider end should be closer to the foot of the bed.
   (C) The wider end should be facing the side of the bed.
   (D) The narrower end should be closer to the head of the bed.

4. Which of the following is a type of elimination equipment used for people who cannot lift their buttocks onto a standard bedpan?
   (A) Portable commode
   (B) Urinal
   (C) Toilet
   (D) Fracture pan

7. Discuss common disorders of the gastrointestinal system

Matching
Use each letter only once.

1. _____ Constipation

2. _____ Crohn's disease

3. _____ Diarrhea

4. _____ Diverticulitis

5. _____ Diverticulosis

6. ____ Fecal impaction

7. ____ Fecal incontinence

8. ____ Flatulence

9. ____ Gastroesophageal reflux disease (GERD)

10. ____ Heartburn

11. ____ Hemorrhoids

12. ____ Irritable bowel syndrome

13. ____ Malabsorption

14. ____ Ulcerative colitis

15. ____ Ulcers

(A) Causes the lining of the digestive tract to become inflamed

(B) Frequent elimination of liquid or semiliquid feces

(C) Results from a weakening of the sphincter muscle that joins the esophagus and the stomach; also known as *acid reflux*

(D) Enlarged veins in the rectum that can cause itching, burning, pain, and bleeding

(E) Raw sores in the stomach and small intestine

(F) Sac-like pouchings develop in weakened areas of the wall of the large intestine (colon)

(G) Chronic condition of the large intestine that is worsened by stress

(H) Chronic condition in which the liquid contents of the stomach back up into the esophagus

(I) Mass of dry, hard stool that remains packed in the rectum and cannot be expelled

(J) Condition in which the body cannot absorb or digest a particular nutrient properly

(K) Inability to control the muscles of the bowels, leading to involuntary passage of stool or gas

(L) Inflammation of and sores in the lining of the large intestine (colon)

(M) Inflammation of sacs that develop in the wall of the large intestine due to diverticulosis

(N) Inability to eliminate stool, or the infrequent, difficult, and often painful elimination of a hard, dry stool

(O) Air in the intestine that is passed through the rectum

8. Discuss how enemas are given

Fill in the Blank

1. An enema is given when help is needed _____ stool from the colon.

2. Enemas are also ordered in preparation for a(n) _____ or _____.

3. _____ water, _____, and _____ enemas are considered cleansing enemas.

4. During the enema, the resident should be in the _____ position.

5. When giving an enema, the nursing assistant should stop immediately if the resident has _____ or if the NA feels resistance.

6. The goals of using an oil-retention enema include lubricating the intestine, softening _____, and reducing _____ with bowel movements.

9. Demonstrate how to collect a stool specimen

True or False

1. ____ A specimen is a sample used for analysis and diagnosis.

2. ____ Blood is one substance for which stool may be tested.

3. ____ If stool needs to be tested for ova and parasites, the NA should place the specimen on ice before taking it to the lab.

4. ____ Specimens are generally stored in the same refrigerators that are used for food and drinks.

5. ____ Urine and toilet paper should not be included in a stool specimen.

6. ____ A plastic collection container called a "hat" is sometimes inserted into a toilet to collect and measure urine or stool.

7. ____ A specimen cannot be collected if a resident is in isolation.

10. Explain occult blood testing

Short Answer

1. How may hidden (occult) blood be detected in stool?

_____

_____

_____

_____

_____

_____

2. Before performing an occult blood test on a stool specimen, what should the nursing assistant check?

_____

_____

_____

_____

_____

11. Define *ostomy* and identify the difference between ileostomy and colostomy

Multiple Choice

1. The surgical creation of an opening from an area inside the body to the outside is called a(n)
   (A) Operation
   (B) Ostomy
   (C) Pouch
   (D) Barrier

2. When a resident has a colostomy, stool will generally be
   (A) Hard
   (B) Semisolid
   (C) Liquid
   (D) Black

3. What is worn over a stoma to collect feces when a resident has an ostomy?
   (A) Disposable pouch
   (B) Biohazard bag
   (C) Surgical netting
   (D) Special backpack

4. When giving ostomy care, in which direction should the nursing assistant wash?
   (A) Toward the stoma
   (B) Away from the stoma
   (C) Into the opening
   (D) In circles

12. Explain guidelines for assisting with bowel retraining

Crossword Puzzle

Across

3. The process of assisting residents to regain control of their bowels or bladder

5. The opposite of negative

6. Can be offered at specific times each day

7. Nursing assistants must answer these promptly during the retraining process

Down

1. Wearing gloves while handling body wastes is a part of these guidelines

2. Predict bathroom times by observing these

4. Providing this as needed helps promote proper hygiene

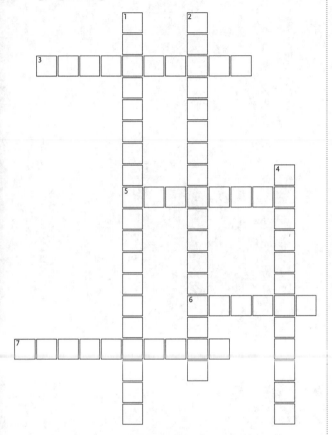

2. Care facilities will have bariatric equipment available, such as the following:
   (A) Sturdier bedpan
   (B) Longer axillary thermometer
   (C) Thick-handled writing utensil
   (D) Separate dining area

3. To prevent complications after surgery, a resident who is obese may require
   (A) Supplemental oxygen
   (B) Less personal care
   (C) Anesthesia that lasts several days following surgery
   (D) Bariatric warm compresses

13. Discuss bariatrics and related care

Multiple Choice

1. To safely transfer a resident who is obese,
   (A) One caregiver with specialized training is required.
   (B) At least two caregivers are required.
   (C) The resident's family must be available to help.
   (D) Two nurses are required.

16

The Urinary System

1. Review the key terms in Learning Objective 1 before completing the workbook exercises

2. Explain the structure and function of the urinary system

Fill in the Blank

1. The urinary system consists of two
_____, two
_____, the urinary bladder, the urethra, and the meatus.

2. Substances not needed by the body—toxins and waste products   stay in the kidneys and form _____.

3. The female urethra is
_____
than the male urethra.

4. The functions of the urinary system are elimination of _____ products from the blood, maintenance of
_____
balance in the body, regulation of the levels of electrolytes in the body, and assistance in regulation of blood pressure.

3. Discuss changes in the urinary system due to aging

True or False

1. _____ Kidneys not filtering blood as efficiently is a normal change of aging.

2. _____ As people age, the bladder holds more urine than it used to.

3. _____ Bladder muscle tone weakens with age.

4. _____ The bladder may not empty completely as a person ages, increasing the chance of infection.

4. List normal qualities of urine and identify signs and symptoms to report about urine

Multiple Choice

1. What should normal urine look like?
(A) It should be cloudy.
(B) It should be pale yellow.
(C) It should be dark brown.
(D) It should be light red.

2. How many milliliters (mL) of urine do adults normally produce per day?
(A) 900 to 1000 mL
(B) 500 to 1000 mL
(C) 200 to 400 mL
(D) 1200 to 1500 mL

3. Which of the following statements is true of urine and urination?
(A) People urinate several times a day to remain healthy.
(B) Urinary incontinence is a normal part of getting older.
(C) People normally urinate twice a day to remain healthy.
(D) Burning during urination is to be expected as a person ages.

5. List factors affecting urination and describe how to promote normal urination

Short Answer

List one way each of these factors affects urination: growth and development, psychological factors, fluid intake, physical activity and exercise, personal habits, medications, and disorders.

_____

_____

_____

_____

_____

_____

_____

_____

_____

_____

_____

_____

_____

_____

_____

_____

_____

_____

_____

_____

6. Discuss common disorders of the urinary system

Matching
Use each letter only once.

1. ____ Chronic renal failure (CRF)

2. ____ Dialysis

3. ____ End-stage renal disease (ESRD)

4. ____ Urinary tract infection (UTI)

5. ____ Urine retention

(A) Artificial means of removing the body's waste products when the kidneys are no longer able to perform this function

(B) Inability to adequately or completely empty the bladder

(C) Progressive condition in which the kidneys cannot effectively filter waste products from the blood

(D) Most common cause of this infection is *E. coli* bacteria

(E) Condition in which kidneys have failed and dialysis or transplantation is required to sustain life

7. Discuss reasons for incontinence

Multiple Choice

1. Urinary incontinence is
   (A) Contagious
   (B) Not a normal part of aging
   (C) Controlled by a low-sodium diet
   (D) A symptom of a healthcare-associated infection

2. Which of the following is a cause of stress incontinence?
   (A) Sneezing
   (B) Drinking too much water
   (C) Weight loss
   (D) High-iron diet

3. Which of the following scenarios describes professional behavior by the NA when dealing with an episode of incontinence?
   (A) As the NA changes the resident's sheets and clothing, she tells the resident that in the future she should press the call light sooner if she needs to use the bathroom.
   (B) The NA steps from the resident's room into the hallway and calls out to her coworkers, "Can somebody please help me? Mrs. Miller wet the bed again."
   (C) The NA changes the resident's undergarment and bed protector and then moves the resident to the side of the bed to let the bottom sheet dry.
   (D) A resident's son presses the call light to report that his father has been incontinent. The NA thanks the son, says she will take care of it right away, and suggests he grab a quick coffee as she begins to gather clean linen and supplies.

4. What can the NA do to reduce or prevent episodes of incontinence?
   (A) The NA should remove the water pitcher from the resident's room.
   (B) The NA should insist that the resident use the toilet before beginning an activity.
   (C) The NA should threaten to use incontinence briefs if the resident does not "hold it."
   (D) The NA should follow the resident's elimination schedule.

5. Which of the following is true of incontinence briefs?
   (A) They come in only one size.
   (B) They are commonly referred to as "diapers" by the care team.
   (C) The NA should check the brief at least every two hours.
   (D) The NA should wash the brief once it is soiled and then reapply it.

8. Describe catheters and related care

Multiple Choice

1. A catheter that remains in the bladder for a period of time is called a(n)
   (A) Straight catheter
   (B) Indwelling catheter
   (C) Condom catheter
   (D) Texas catheter

2. What is the nursing assistant's role regarding catheters?
   (A) Giving daily catheter care
   (B) Inserting the catheter
   (C) Irrigating the catheter
   (D) Removing the catheter

3. Which of the following statements is true of providing catheter care?
   (A) The nursing assistant should give daily care of the genital area to keep it clean.
   (B) The nursing assistant should make sure the drainage bag hangs higher than the level of the hips or bladder.
   (C) The nursing assistant should store the drainage bag on the floor.
   (D) The nursing assistant should reattach the catheter tube if it disconnects.

4. When providing catheter care, how much of the catheter tubing should the nursing assistant clean?
   (A) At least two inches
   (B) At least four inches
   (C) At least six inches
   (D) At least eight inches

5. A catheter that is inserted to drain urine from the bladder several times a day and is removed each time after urine is drained is called a(n)
   (A) Straight catheter
   (B) Indwelling catheter
   (C) Condom catheter
   (D) Texas catheter

Name: _____

9. Explain how to collect different types of urine specimens

Matching
Use each letter only once.

1. _____ 24-hour urine specimen

2. _____ Catheterized urine specimen

3. _____ Clean-catch urine specimen

4. _____ Routine urine specimen

(A) Collects all urine voided by resident during a 24-hour period

(B) First and last urine voided is not included in the sample

(C) May be done when a resident has urinary retention

(D) Can be collected any time resident voids

10. Explain types of tests that are performed on urine

Multiple Choice

1. Chemical substances produced when the body burns fat for energy or fuel may be found in urine when a person has diabetes. These substances are called
   (A) Particles
   (B) Glucose
   (C) Ketones
   (D) pH levels

2. How do reagent strips show the result of a urine test?
   (A) They change color when they react with urine.
   (B) They disintegrate when they react with urine.
   (C) They become rigid when they react with urine.
   (D) They break into small pieces when they react with urine.

3. Using the pH scale, which of the following numbers would show that the urine is more acidic (as opposed to alkaline)?
   (A) 5
   (B) 6
   (C) 7
   (D) 8

4. What kind of test evaluates the body's water balance and urine concentration by showing how the density of urine compares with water?
   (A) Occult blood test
   (B) Glucose level test
   (C) pH level test
   (D) Specific gravity test

11. Explain guidelines for assisting with bladder retraining

True or False

1. _____ Loss of normal bladder function can be caused by illness, injury, or inactivity.

2. _____ Residents will not usually be embarrassed by episodes of incontinence.

3. _____ Observing residents' elimination habits helps predict when a trip to the bathroom may be necessary.

4. _____ The nursing assistant should offer a trip to the bathroom, bedpan, or urinal before beginning procedures and after completing procedures.

5. _____ Residents who have problems with incontinence should be discouraged from drinking fluids.

6. _____ If a nursing assistant can let the resident know how frustrated she is when the resident is incontinent, it will encourage him to control his bladder.

7. _____ Residents must be encouraged to ask for help with elimination whenever they need it.

17

The Reproductive System

1. Review the key terms in Learning Objective 1 before completing the workbook exercises

2. Explain the structure and function of the reproductive system

Fill in the Blank

1. Ova are released from the ovaries each month during the process of
_____.

2. The male and female reproductive glands are called _____.

3. The female reproductive system produces the female sex cells and the female hormones _____ and _____.

4. The female reproductive system is made up of the _____, fallopian tubes, uterus, _____, the vulva, and the breasts.

5. The male reproductive system consists of the _____, testes, scrotum, epididymis, vas deferens, _____ tissue, seminal vesicle, ejaculatory duct, and _____ gland.

6. If an ovum is fertilized, it moves into the
_____.

7. The male reproductive system produces the male hormone _____.

8. Every milliliter of semen contains 20 to 150 million _____.

3. Discuss changes in the reproductive system due to aging

True or False

1. _____ A man's prostate gland enlarges with age.

2. _____ Menopause is a normal change of aging.

3. _____ A woman's production of estrogen and progesterone increases as she ages.

4. _____ Number and capability of sperm decrease with age.

5. _____ It takes less time for an older man to achieve an erection and to reach orgasm.

6. _____ As a woman ages, her vaginal walls become drier and thinner, which may cause discomfort during sexual intercourse.

4. Discuss common disorders of the reproductive system

Matching
For each of the following descriptions, write the letter of the disorder to which it refers. Use each letter only once.

1. _____ Benign prostatic hypertrophy

2. _____ Chlamydia

3. _____ Genital herpes

4. _____ Genital HPV infection

5. _____ Gonorrhea

6. ____ Syphilis

7. ____ Trichomoniasis

8. ____ Vaginitis

(A) The prostate becomes enlarged and causes problems with urination

(B) Bacterial infection that causes burning with urination, discharge from the penis or vagina, and lower back pain

(C) Caused by a virus and cannot be cured; symptoms include itching and painful red blisters or open sores

(D) Inflammation of the vagina that causes vaginal discharge, itching, and pain

(E) Green, cloudy, pus-like discharge from the penis and swollen testes; can cause sterility and pelvic inflammatory disease if not treated

(F) Caused by a virus; genital warts may appear

(G) Bacterial infection that may cause small, painless sores to appear on the penis soon after infection

(H) Caused by protozoa; symptoms include a green-yellow vaginal discharge with a strong odor

5. Describe sexual needs of the elderly

Short Answer

1. What is true of sexual needs as a person ages?

_____

_____

_____

_____

_____

_____

_____

_____

_____

2. What should a nursing assistant do if she encounters consenting adult residents in a sexual situation?

_____

_____

_____

18

The Integumentary System

1. Review the key terms in Learning Objective 1 before completing the workbook exercises

2. Explain the structure and function of the integumentary system

Fill in the Blank

1. The skin is the largest _____ in the human body.

2. The substance that gives skin its color is _____.

3. The skin covers and _____ the body, provides _____ through nerves, regulates body temperature, and prevents the loss of too much _____.

4. The two basic layers of the skin are the _____ and the _____.

5. _____ are found in the skin and give the ability to feel and touch.

Short Answer

1. List the parts of the integumentary system.

_____

_____

_____

_____

_____

_____

2. List five functions of the integumentary system.

_____

_____

_____

_____

_____

_____

_____

_____

_____

_____

3. Discuss changes in the integumentary system due to aging

True or False

1. ____ Skin cancer occurs normally as a person ages.

2. ____ The amount of fat and collagen increases with age.

3. ____ Skin loses elasticity with age, causing wrinkles.

4. ____ Skin becoming thinner and more fragile is a normal change of aging.

5. ____ Nail growth slows as a person ages.

6. ____ Brown spots may appear on the skin in areas exposed to the sun.

7. ____ Hair becoming thicker is a normal change of aging.

4. Discuss common disorders of the integumentary system

Matching
Use each letter only once.

1. ____ Burns

2. ____ Cellulitis

3. ____ Dermatitis

4. ____ Fungal infections

5. ____ Gangrene

6. ____ Psoriasis

7. ____ Scabies

8. ____ Shingles

9. ____ Skin cancer

10. ____ Warts

11. ____ Wounds

(A) Caused by tiny mites that burrow into the skin to lay eggs

(B) Death of tissue caused by a lack of blood flow

(C) Rough, hard bumps caused by a virus that invades the skin, usually through a cut or tear

(D) Chronic skin condition in which cells of the skin grow too fast, causing red, white, or silver patches to form

(E) Commonly occurs in moist areas, such as under the breasts and in the groin area; yeast is one type

(F) Can be classified as superficial, partial-thickness, and full-thickness

(G) Caused by the same virus that causes chickenpox

(H) Inflammation of the skin

(I) An infection of the skin that occurs when bacteria move deeper into the tissues; commonly caused by a break in the skin

(J) Growth of abnormal skin cells; most serious form is malignant melanoma

(K) Types of these include abrasions, avulsions, incisions, lacerations, and punctures

5. Discuss pressure injuries and identify prevention guidelines

Multiple Choice

1. Where does skin breakdown usually occur?
   (A) At pressure points
   (B) On the hands
   (C) On the nose
   (D) Underneath facial hair

2. Areas of the body where the bone lies close to the skin are called bony prominences. An example of a bony prominence where pressure injuries are likely to occur is
   (A) The hands
   (B) The heels
   (C) The forearms
   (D) The eyes

3. What conditions commonly contribute to skin breakdown?
   (A) Moisture and being confined to bed
   (B) A cool and dry environment
   (C) Clean skin and being ambulatory
   (D) Cold air and cold surfaces

4. During the first stage of a pressure injury, skin appears
   (A) Yellow-streaked
   (B) Blue
   (C) Nonintact
   (D) A different color than the surrounding area

5. At a minimum, how often should nursing assistants help immobile residents to change position?
   (A) Every 30 minutes
   (B) Every hour
   (C) Every two hours
   (D) Twice per day

6. Explain the benefits of warm and cold applications

True or False

1. ____ Warm or cold applications can be either moist or dry.

2. ____ The body responds to both heat and cold in the same way.

3. ____ Warm applications close blood vessels, and cold applications open them.

4. ____ A nursing assistant should always wear gloves when helping with a sitz bath.

5. ____ Moist applications are less likely to cause injury than dry applications.

6. ____ Residents with high temperatures may need to have a cooling or tepid sponge bath.

7. ____ Warm and cold applications should not be applied for more than 20 minutes at a time.

Multiple Choice

1. Benefits of using heat include
   (A) Relieving pain and muscular tension
   (B) Decreasing blood flow to the area
   (C) Stopping bleeding
   (D) Constricting/closing blood vessels

2. Benefits of using cold include
   (A) Dilating/opening blood vessels
   (B) Increasing blood flow to the area
   (C) Stopping bleeding
   (D) Making skin cyanotic

3. How does moisture affect warm and cold applications?
   (A) Moisture strengthens the effect of heat and cold.
   (B) Moisture weakens the effect of heat and cold.
   (C) Moisture has no effect.
   (D) Moisture allows use of warm and cold applications for longer than 20 minutes.

4. Which of the following is true of sitz baths?
   (A) Sitz baths are often ordered to help relieve back pain and tension.
   (B) Sitz baths are given with the resident standing up.
   (C) Sitz baths can cause the resident to feel weak and dizzy.
   (D) Sitz baths are used for swelling of the feet and hands.

7. Discuss nonsterile and sterile dressings

Short Answer

1. How do open wounds increase the risk of infection?

   _____

   _____

   _____

   _____

   _____

2. When are nonsterile dressings applied to wounds? When are sterile dressings applied to wounds?

   _____

   _____

   _____

   _____

   _____

   _____

   _____

   _____

The Integumentary System

3. List three types of supplies that are considered sterile.

   _____

   _____

   _____

   _____

   _____

   _____

   _____

   _____

4. What happens if any part of a sterile field becomes contaminated?

   _____

   _____

   _____

   _____

   _____

   _____

   _____

   _____

   _____

19

The Circulatory or Cardiovascular System

1. Review the key terms in Learning Objective 1 before completing the workbook exercises

2. Explain the structure and function of the circulatory system

Multiple Choice

1. What is the pump of the circulatory system?
    (A) Lymph
    (B) Lungs
    (C) Blood vessels
    (D) Heart

2. Which of the following is the phase during which the heart rests?
    (A) Systole
    (B) Diastole
    (C) Ventricle
    (D) Atrical

3. Plasma is made up of mostly
    (A) Blood
    (B) Water
    (C) Lymph
    (D) Marrow

4. Carbon dioxide is removed in the lungs when a person
    (A) Inhales
    (B) Exhales
    (C) Holds his breath
    (D) Eats

5. Blood is made up of solids and liquids:
    (A) Cells and plasma
    (B) Oxygen and lymph
    (C) Potassium and oxygen
    (D) Salt and water

6. What do platelets cause the blood to do?
    (A) Clot
    (B) Move
    (C) Stop
    (D) Feed

7. The largest artery in the body is the
    (A) Carotid
    (B) Vena cava
    (C) Aorta
    (D) Thymus

8. _____ gives blood its red color.
    (A) Salt
    (B) Iron
    (C) B12
    (D) Plasma

3. Discuss changes in the circulatory system due to aging

True or False

1. ____ Heart disease is a normal part of aging.

2. ____ The heart pumping less efficiently is a normal part of aging.

3. ____ Blood vessels widen with age.

4. ____ Blood vessels become less elastic as a person ages.

5. ____ As a person gets older, blood flow increases.

4. Discuss common disorders of the circulatory system

Matching
Use each letter only once.

1. ____ Anemia

2. ____ Angina pectoris

3. ____ Congestive heart failure (CHF)

4. ____ Coronary artery disease (CAD)

5. ____ Deep vein thrombosis (DVT)

6. ____ Elastic stockings

7. ____ Hypertension (HTN)

8. ____ Myocardial infarction (MI, heart attack)

9. ____ Orthopnea

10. ____ Peripheral vascular disease (PVD)

11. ____ Stable angina

12. ____ Sudden cardiac arrest (SCA)

13. ____ Unstable angina

(A) Condition in which the coronary arteries become damaged and narrow over time, causing chest pain and other symptoms

(B) Condition in which the amount of red blood cells or hemoglobin in the body is less than normal

(C) Help increase blood circulation, reduce fluid retention, and prevent an embolism

(D) All or part of the blood flow to the heart muscle is blocked, causing muscle cells to die

(E) Condition in which the blood supply to the legs, feet, arms, or hands is decreased due to poor circulation

(F) Chest pain, pressure, or discomfort due to coronary artery disease

(G) Shortness of breath when lying down that is relieved by sitting up

(H) Condition that occurs when the heart muscle fails to pump effectively, causing a variety of symptoms, including fatigue and the reduced ability to exercise or be active

(I) Chest pain that occurs when a person is active or under severe stress

(J) Chest pain that occurs when a person is at rest and not exerting himself

(K) Blood pressure consistently measuring 130/80 mm Hg or higher

(L) Condition often caused by an arrhythmia in which the heart suddenly stops beating, breathing stops, and consciousness is lost

(M) Condition in which a blood clot forms in a large vein in the body, most often in the leg

20

The Respiratory System

1. Review the key terms in Learning Objective 1 before completing the workbook exercises

2. Explain the structure and function of the respiratory system

Fill in the Blank

1. Two functions of the respiratory system are to _____ oxygen to body cells and _____ carbon dioxide from the cells.

2. _____ is the process that consists of inspiration (inhaling) and expiration (exhaling).

3. The epiglottis blocks food from entering the windpipe, or _____.

4. The _____ expand and contract the chest cavity during _____, when a person breathes in.

5. The larynx enables _____.

6. The lungs are covered by a membrane called the _____.

7. The exchange of _____ and _____ gases occurs in the lungs and in the cells.

8. The process of breathing air in and out is _____; it never stops.

9. The air sacs of the lungs are called the _____.

Short Answer

1. List the parts of the respiratory system.

    _____

    _____

    _____

    _____

    _____

    _____

    _____

    _____

    _____

    _____

2. List the four functions of the respiratory system.

    _____

    _____

    _____

    _____

    _____

    _____

    _____

    _____

3. Discuss changes in the respiratory system due to aging

True or False

1. ____   A decrease in lung capacity is a normal change of aging.

2. _____ Asthma is a normal part of aging.

3. _____ As a person ages, the air sacs in the lungs become less elastic and decrease in number.

4. _____ Airways become more elastic with age, increasing movement of air inside the lungs.

5. _____ When a person gets older, his chest muscles become weaker.

6. _____ With age, the cough reflex becomes more effective, and coughs become stronger.

7. _____ Oxygen in the blood decreases with age.

8. _____ A person's voice becomes weaker as she gets older.

4. Discuss common disorders of the respiratory system

Matching
Use each letter only once.

1. _____ Acute bronchitis

2. _____ Asthma

3. _____ Bronchiectasis

4. _____ Chronic bronchitis

5. _____ Chronic obstructive pulmonary disease (COPD)

6. _____ Emphysema

7. _____ Multidrug-resistant TB (MDR-TB)

8. _____ Pneumonia

9. _____ Tuberculosis (TB)

(A) Type of bronchitis caused by an infection; usually treated with antibiotics

(B) Highly contagious airborne disease that usually affects the lungs, but may affect other parts of the body; causes coughing, difficulty breathing, and fatigue

(C) Chronic, progressive disease leading to difficulty breathing due to obstruction of the airways

(D) Chronic, episodic disorder causing difficulty breathing, heavy wheezing, coughing, and a tight feeling in the chest

(E) Chronic condition that usually results from cigarette smoking and chronic bronchitis

(F) Form of tuberculosis caused by an organism that is resistant to medication that is used to treat TB

(G) Permanent dilation/widening of the bronchi that causes chronic coughing, shortness of breath, weight loss, and coughing up blood

(H) Type of bronchitis in which the lining of bronchial tubes becomes inflamed, causing coughing and restricted air flow

(I) Inflammation of the lungs caused by viral, bacterial, or fungal infection or chemical irritants

5. Describe oxygen delivery

True or False

1. _____ Nursing assistants may adjust a resident's oxygen levels if the resident requests it.

2. _____ It is safe to smoke around oxygen, as long as it is not done within three feet of the oxygen device.

3. _____ Oxygen therapy is the administration of oxygen to increase the supply of oxygen to the lungs.

4. _____ The nursing assistant should turn off the oxygen delivery device if the equipment does not seem to be working.

5. _____ Common types of oxygen delivery devices include the nasal cannula, simple face mask, and the oxygen concentrator.

6. _____ It is important for the nursing assistant to perform frequent skin care on areas of the face on which an oxygen device rests.

7. _____ Petroleum-based lubricants are best for soothing sensitive areas on the nose and mouth when a person is using oxygen.

8. ____ A nursing assistant should encourage activity as permitted for residents who are receiving oxygen.

9. ____ The nursing assistant should report sores on the nasal area to the nurse.

10. ____ All residents using oxygen will need oxygen continuously.

6. Describe how to collect a sputum specimen

Crossword Puzzle

Across

5. Best time of the day to collect sputum

6. Comes from the salivary glands and is not the same as sputum

Down

1. One of the things that a sputum specimen is checked for

2. Mucus that comes from inside the respiratory system

3. Liquid used to rinse the mouth before obtaining a sputum specimen

4. Fluid that should not be used for rinsing the mouth before a sputum collection

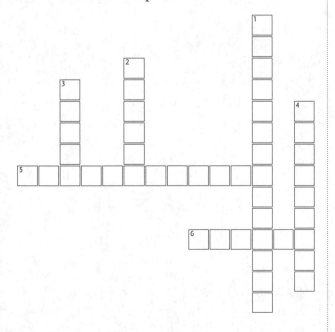

7. Describe the benefits of deep breathing exercises

Multiple Choice

1. When a resident is using an incentive spirometer, what kind of breathing should he do?
   (A) Shallow breathing
   (B) Fast breathing
   (C) Short breathing
   (D) Deep breathing

2. What is the first step the nursing assistant should take before helping a resident with an incentive spirometer?
   (A) The NA should wash her hands.
   (B) The NA should don gloves.
   (C) The NA should don a gown.
   (D) The NA should place the mouthpiece in the resident's mouth.

3. What is one of the nursing assistant's responsibilities regarding the incentive spirometer?
   (A) The NA should administer lung medication via an inhaler before the resident uses the device.
   (B) The NA should encourage the resident to take a deep breath while using the device.
   (C) The NA should insist that the resident use the device even if the resident does not want to do so.
   (D) The NA should make sure the device remains on its side while the resident is using it.

Name: _____

21

The Musculoskeletal System

1. Review the key terms in Learning Objective 1 before completing the workbook exercises

2. Explain the structure and function of the musculoskeletal system

Fill in the Blank

1. The musculoskeletal system gives the body _____ and _____.

2. The musculoskeletal system allows the body to _____ and _____ itself, provides _____ for the body, and creates _____.

3. Muscles are groups of _____ that help the body move by _____ and _____.

4. _____ are the rigid connective tissues that make up the _____, which is the framework of the human body.

5. _____ are found at the place where two bones come together; they hold bones together and provide movement and _____.

6. _____ are strong, fibrous bands that connect bones or cartilage and help _____ the joints and joint movement.

Short Answer

1. List the five parts of the musculoskeletal system.

    _____

    _____

    _____

    _____

    _____

    _____

    _____

    _____

2. List the three types of muscles in the body.

    _____

    _____

    _____

    _____

    _____

    _____

    _____

3. List the four types of bones.

    _____

    _____

    _____

    _____

_____
_____
_____
_____
_____

4. List the seven functions of the musculoskeletal system.

_____
_____
_____
_____
_____
_____
_____
_____
_____
_____
_____
_____
_____

3. Discuss changes in the musculoskeletal system due to aging

True or False

1. ____ As people age, the body loses muscle mass.

2. ____ As people age, the amount of calcium in the bones increases.

3. ____ Bones are more easily broken as people age.

4. ____ Joints become more flexible with age.

5. ____ As people age, height is gradually lost.

4. Discuss common disorders of the musculoskeletal system

Matching
Use each letter only once.

1. ____ Amputation

2. ____ Arthritis

3. ____ Bursitis

4. ____ Fibromyalgia syndrome

5. ____ Fracture

6. ____ Muscular dystrophy

7. ____ Osteoarthritis

8. ____ Osteopenia

9. ____ Osteoporosis

10. ____ Phantom limb pain

11. ____ Phantom sensation

12. ____ Prosthesis

13. ____ Rheumatoid arthritis

14. ____ Total hip replacement

15. ____ Total knee replacement

16. ____ Traction

(A) Condition in which bones lose density, causing them to be brittle and easily broken

(B) Surgical removal of part or all of a body part

(C) Surgical replacement of a knee with artificial
materials

(D) An artificial device that replaces a body part,
such as an eye, tooth, arm, leg, hip, or heart
valve

(E) Surgical replacement of the head of the
femur and the socket it fits into where it
joins the hip

(F) General term for inflammation of the joints
that can cause pain, stiffness, and swelling

(G) Condition in which the small sacs of fluid
near the joints become inflamed

(H) Hereditary, progressive disease that causes muscles to weaken and stiffen, and hands and arms to twitch

(I) Condition that affects the synovial membrane and causes stiffness, swelling, severe pain, and deformities that can be severe and disabling

(J) Feeling of pain in a limb or extremity that has been amputated

(K) Feeling of warmth, itching, and tingling in the area where a limb was amputated

(L) Condition in which the cushiony cartilage that rests between the bones and pads the ends of the bones begins to slowly erode, causing pain, redness, swelling, and stiffness

(M) A broken bone

(N) Method of treating fractures that keeps bones in the proper position by using weights and pulleys

(O) Disorder that causes pain, fatigue, sleep problems, problems with thinking and memory, and depression

(P) Condition in which bones lose density but not enough density to be classified as osteoporosis

Short Answer

1. List five guidelines for cast care.

_____

_____

_____

_____

_____

_____

_____

_____

2. List six guidelines for care of a resident who is recovering from a total hip replacement.

_____

_____

_____

_____

_____

_____

_____

_____

_____

_____

_____

_____

_____

_____

_____

3. Define these terms: partial weight-bearing (PWB), non-weight-bearing (NWB), and full weight-bearing (FWB).

_____

_____

_____

_____

_____

_____

_____

_____

_____

_____

_____

Name: _____

5. Describe elastic bandages

Multiple Choice

1. Another name for an elastic bandage is a(n)
   (A) Nonsterile bandage
   (B) Band-aid
   (C) Surgical bandage
   (D) Abdominal binder

2. What is one reason that elastic bandages are used?
   (A) To keep a broken bone in the proper position for healing
   (B) To provide compression and support for body parts
   (C) To keep skin warm and dry
   (D) To treat pressure injuries in advanced stages

3. Elastic bandages should be wrapped in a _____ direction.
   (A) Clean to dirty
   (B) Front to back
   (C) Far to near
   (D) Intact to nonintact

22

The Nervous System

1. Review the key terms in Learning Objective 1 before completing the workbook exercises

2. Explain the structure and function of the nervous system

Fill in the Blank

1. The nervous system _____ and _____ all body functions.

2. The nervous system also _____ and _____ information from outside the body.

3. The _____ is the basic working unit of the nervous system.

4. The two main parts of the nervous system are the _____ nervous system and the _____ nervous system.

5. The peripheral nervous system consists of the _____ and _____ nerves.

6. The _____ and _____ make up the central nervous system.

7. The ear provides _____ and _____.

8. The nervous system provides _____ centers for heartbeat and respiration.

9. The sense organs are part of the nervous system. They include the _____, tongue, _____, eyes, and _____.

10. Inside the back of the eye is the _____, which contains cells that respond to light and send messages to the brain.

3. Discuss changes in the nervous system due to aging

True or False

1. ____ Weakened vision is a normal part of aging.

2. ____ Some short-term memory loss may occur with age.

3. ____ As people age, the senses normally become stronger.

4. ____ Responses and reflexes speed up with age.

5. ____ Sensitivity of nerve endings decreases with age, resulting in diminished sense of touch.

6. ____ Slight hearing loss is not a normal change of aging.

4. Discuss common disorders of the nervous system

Matching
Use each letter only once.

1. ____ Age-related macular degeneration

2. ____ Cataract

Name: _____

3. _____ Cerebrovascular accident (CVA)

4. _____ Concussion

5. _____ Dysphagia

6. _____ Emotional lability

7. _____ Epilepsy

8. _____ Expressive aphasia

9. _____ Farsightedness (hyperopia)

10. _____ Glaucoma

11. _____ Hemiparesis

12. _____ Hemiplegia

13. _____ Meniere's disease

14. _____ Multiple sclerosis (MS)

15. _____ Nearsightedness (myopia)

16. _____ One-sided neglect

17. _____ Otitis media

18. _____ Paraplegia

19. _____ Parkinson's disease

20. _____ Quadriplegia

21. _____ Receptive aphasia

22. _____ Transient ischemic attack (TIA)

(A) Paralysis on one side of the body

(B) Loss of function of the lower body and legs

(C) Disorder that causes recurring seizures

(D) Disorder of the inner ear caused by fluid buildup

(E) Difficulty swallowing

(F) Condition that causes the part of the retina that allows people to see detail to degenerate, destroying central vision

(G) Difficulty understanding spoken or written words

(H) An infection of the middle ear that causes pain, pressure, fever, and reduced ability to hear

(I) The pressure inside the eye increases, causing damage to the optic nerve

(J) Develops when the lens of the eye becomes cloudy, causing vision loss

(K) Ability to see objects that are near more clearly than distant objects

(L) Progressive disorder that causes loss of the protective covering that protects nerves and spinal cord

(M) Caused by a blockage of the blood supply to the brain or a leaking or ruptured blood vessel within the brain

(N) Difficulty communicating through speech or writing

(O) Tendency to ignore a weak or paralyzed side of the body

(P) Warning sign of a cerebrovascular accident

(Q) Head injury that occurs from a banging movement of the brain against the skull

(R) Progressive disorder that can cause tremors and a mask-like facial expression

(S) Inappropriate or unprovoked emotional responses

(T) Loss of function of the arms, trunk, and legs

(U) Weakness on one side of the body

(V) Ability to see distant objects more clearly than objects that are near

True or False

1. _____ Strokes that occur on the right side of the brain affect functioning on the right side of the body.

2. _____ Diminished awareness or one-sided paralysis causes a lack of sensation that increases the risk of injury.

3. _____ Residents with Parkinson's disease may need to do range of motion exercises to prevent contractures.

4. _____ Multiple sclerosis is often diagnosed in young adulthood.

5. _____ Spinal cord injuries are treated with more success if the cord is completely cut or severed.

6. _____ Eye drops are used to treat glaucoma.

Multiple Choice

1. Which of the following statements is true of a hearing aid?
    (A) A hearing aid should be soaked in warm water before cleaning.
    (B) The hearing aid should be turned off when it is not in use.
    (C) The volume should be turned up just before inserting a hearing aid.
    (D) A hearing aid should remain in the ear when a person is showering.

2. Which of the following statements is true of an artificial eye?
    (A) An artificial eye provides vision.
    (B) An artificial eye should be disinfected with rubbing alcohol.
    (C) An artificial eye is normally stored in a dry cup on a paper towel.
    (D) An artificial eye is held in place by suction.

3. When a resident has a vision impairment, a nursing assistant should
    (A) Use the face of an imaginary clock as a guide to explain the position of items
    (B) Keep the door partially open so that the resident can find the doorway
    (C) Enter the room first before identifying herself, so as not to frighten the resident
    (D) Walk behind the resident, calling out warnings when stairs and steps appear

4. The best way that a nursing assistant can help a resident who has had a stroke is to
    (A) Make sure the resident is constantly doing tasks in order to keep him energized
    (B) Use short, simple sentences when communicating
    (C) Stand on the resident's stronger side when transferring him
    (D) Remind the resident which is his "bad leg" and which is his "good leg" so that he does not get them confused

5. Residents who have paralysis are at a higher risk of injury from
    (A) Heat and cold
    (B) Heart disease
    (C) Drinking too many fluids
    (D) Bowel retraining

5. Discuss dementia and related terms

Multiple Choice

1. Which of the following statements is true of dementia?
    (A) Dementia is the ability to think clearly and logically.
    (B) Dementia is a normal change of aging in the brain.
    (C) Dementia is a serious loss of mental abilities that interferes with normal functioning.
    (D) Dementia is an increase in cognitive abilities.

2. The most common form of dementia is
    (A) Parkinson's disease
    (B) AIDS
    (C) Alzheimer's disease
    (D) Huntington's disease

3. Which of the following statements is true of dementia?
    (A) Most forms of dementia are reversible.
    (B) Nutritional deficiencies are the most common cause of dementia.
    (C) Making a diagnosis of dementia is difficult.
    (D) Dementia is commonly caused by getting older.

6. Discuss Alzheimer's disease and identify its stages

Short Answer

1. Define *Alzheimer's disease*.

    _____

    _____

    _____

Name: _____

_____

_____

_____

_____

_____

_____

2. Briefly describe what occurs in each of the three stages of Alzheimer's disease.

Mild Alzheimer's disease

_____

_____

_____

_____

_____

_____

_____

_____

_____

Moderate Alzheimer's disease

_____

_____

_____

_____

_____

_____

_____

_____

_____

Severe Alzheimer's disease

_____

_____

_____

_____

_____

_____

_____

_____

_____

_____

_____

_____

3. Why is it important to encourage independence in residents with Alzheimer's disease?

_____

_____

_____

_____

7. List strategies for better communication with residents with Alzheimer's disease

Crossword Puzzle

Across

1. A nursing assistant should limit the times she uses this word and instead should redirect activities

4. The repetition of words, phrases, and actions

Down

2. Types of cues to observe as the ability to talk lessens

3. A nursing assistant should first

   _____

   herself when greeting a resident with Alzheimer's disease

5. Talking about only one of these at a time while using simple, short sentences may be helpful when dealing with a resident with Alzheimer's disease

6. An example of nonverbal communication that can be used as speaking abilities decline

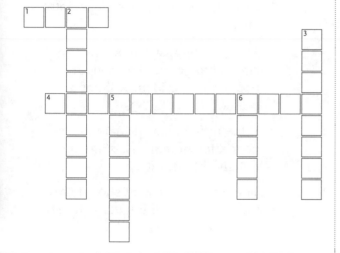

8. Identify personal attitudes helpful in caring for residents with Alzheimer's disease

Short Answer
For each of the helpful attitudes listed, write one reason why it is important.

1. Do not take things personally.

   _____

   _____

   _____

   _____

   _____

   _____

   _____

2. Be empathetic.

   _____

   _____

   _____

   _____

   _____

   _____

   _____

   _____

3. Work with the symptoms and behaviors noted.

   _____

   _____

   _____

   _____

   _____

   _____

   _____

4. Work as a team.

   _____

   _____

   _____

   _____

   _____

Name: _____

5. Be aware of difficulties associated with caregiving.

_____

_____

_____

_____

_____

_____

_____

6. Work with family members.

_____

_____

_____

_____

_____

_____

_____

_____

_____

7. Remember the goals of the care plan.

_____

_____

_____

_____

_____

_____

_____

_____

_____

9. Describe guidelines for problems with common activities of daily living (ADLs)

True or False

1. ____ Nonslip mats, tub seats, and hand-holds should be used to ensure safety during bathing.

2. ____ The resident should always bathe at the same time every day, even if he is agitated.

3. ____ The nursing assistant should break tasks down into simple steps, introducing one step at a time.

4. ____ The nursing assistant should not attempt to groom the resident because the resident will not understand it.

5. ____ If the resident has urinary incontinence, the nursing assistant should not give him fluids.

6. ____ The nursing assistant should check the resident's skin regularly for signs of irritation.

7. ____ The nursing assistant should choose clothes that are easy to put on.

8. ____ The bathroom should be marked with a sign as a reminder to use it and to show where it is.

9. ____ For mealtime, plain plates with simple place settings should be used.

10. ____ The nursing assistant should not encourage independence, as this leads to aggressive behavior.

11. ____ The resident's weight should be monitored accurately and frequently.

12. ____ The nursing assistant should reward positive behavior with smiles and warm touches.

10. Describe interventions for common difficult behaviors related to Alzheimer's disease

Scenarios
Read each of the following scenarios involving residents with Alzheimer's disease and answer the questions that follow.

1. Dana is a nursing assistant who has just started working at Parkwood Care Facility. She is assigned to give Mr. Gutiérrez, a resident with Alzheimer's disease, a bath and a back rub. When Dana meets Mr. Gutiérrez, he gets very upset and yells at Dana to leave him alone. What can Dana do to lessen Mr. Gutiérrez's agitation?

_____

_____

_____

_____

_____

_____

_____

2. Mr. Aaronson, another resident at Parkwood, is upset because he has just found out that his daughter is moving out of the state and will not be able to visit him as often. While watching television in the common area with other residents, he gets angry at Mrs. Robinson for changing the channel. He starts shouting at her and threatens to hit her if she does not stop irritating him. How should Dana respond to this behavior?

_____

_____

_____

_____

_____

_____

3. Dana notices that one of her residents, Mr. Boyd, has seemed withdrawn lately and has not been eating as much as usual. He has lost interest in his treasured book collection and has not wanted to spend any time with his friends or family when they visit. What can Dana do?

_____

_____

_____

_____

_____

_____

_____

_____

4. When Dana arrives at work one morning, she gets several complaints from her residents that Mr. Gutiérrez has been scratching his groin area in the dining room during breakfast and making the other residents at his table uncomfortable. What are some possible causes for this behavior, and how should Dana react?

_____

_____

_____

_____

_____

_____

5. Ms. Singer is a cheerful, vivacious resident with Alzheimer's disease. She loves to dress in brightly colored clothes and wear tasteful jewelry. Lately she has begun to pick up other residents' clothing and jewelry from their rooms and put them into her dresser drawer. Her family is very upset by this behavior. What should Dana tell them and how can she help?

_____

_____

_____

_____

_____

_____

_____

_____

_____

11. Discuss ways to provide activities for residents with Alzheimer's disease

True or False

1. _____ Residents with Alzheimer's disease usually do not enjoy participating in activities.

2. _____ Information about a resident from his family should be used to plan activities for him.

3. _____ Meaningful activities for a resident with Alzheimer's disease draw on past skills that the resident has used throughout his life.

4. _____ Activities will keep a resident with Alzheimer's disease focused for several hours at a time.

5. _____ If a resident loses interest in an activity, the staff should push her to continue until she is finished because it promotes a healthy self-esteem.

6. _____ Residents' families should be encouraged to participate in activities.

7. _____ Residents with Alzheimer's disease should be discouraged from exercising.

8. _____ Each resident should be encouraged to use her special skills.

9. _____ Reading and playing music are good ways to provide activity for residents who are bedbound.

12. Describe therapies for residents with Alzheimer's disease

Matching
Use each letter only once.

1. _____ Reminiscence therapy

2. _____ Remotivation therapy

3. _____ Validation therapy

(A) Type of therapy that promotes self-esteem, self-awareness, and socialization by having residents gather in small groups

(B) Type of therapy that lets people with Alzheimer's disease believe they live in the past or in imaginary circumstances

(C) Type of therapy that encourages people with Alzheimer's disease to remember and talk about the past

13. Discuss mental health and mental health disorders

Fill in the Blank

1. _____ is a person's ability to use cognition and emotion appropriately.

2. A mental health disorder is a _____ that affects a person's ability to function within family, home, work, or community settings.

3. _____ is characterized by excessive worrying, tension, and unease, even when there is no apparent cause for these feelings.

4. A person who has witnessed or experienced a traumatic event such as being a victim of a crime or being in combat while in the military may develop

_____

_____.

5. Obsessive-compulsive disorder is characterized by _____ behavior or thoughts.

6. _____
disorder causes extreme self-consciousness in common situations and may cause a person to avoid being around other people.

7. _____
_____ is
a type of mental health disorder that causes withdrawal, lack of energy, and apathy.

8. Major depressive disorder is treated with _____ and _____.

9. A person with

_____

_____

may have mood swings and changes in energy level and ability to function.

10. Symptoms of _____ include hallucinations, delusions, and disorganized thinking and speech.

14. Discuss substance abuse and list signs of substance abuse to report

Short Answer

1. What is one reason why opioid abuse is prevalent in the United States.

_____

_____

_____

_____

_____

2. List four risk factors for substance abuse.

_____

_____

_____

_____

_____

_____

3. Under what circumstances is an elderly person more at risk for substance abuse?

_____

_____

_____

_____

_____

_____

_____

Name: _____

23
The Endocrine System

1. Review the key terms in Learning Objective 1 before completing the workbook exercises

2. Explain the structure and function of the endocrine system

Fill in the Blank

1. Glands produce and secrete chemicals called
   _____.

2. The
   _____
   secrete testosterone.

3. The endocrine system is made up of
   _____
   in different areas of the body.

4. The endocrine system influences growth
   and _____,
   maintains blood sugar levels, and regulates
   the ability to
   _____.

5. The _____ gland
   is also referred to as the *master gland*.

6. During stressful situations,
   _____
   and the less potent noradrenaline increase
   the efficiency of muscle contractions,
   increase _____
   rate and blood pressure, and also increase
   blood glucose levels to provide extra energy.

7. The pancreas produces
   _____,
   which regulates the amount of glucose available to the cells for metabolism.

3. Discuss changes in the endocrine system due to aging

True or False

1. ____ Menopause is a normal change of aging in women.

2. ____ As men age, testosterone production stops.

3. ____ Insulin production increases with age.

4. ____ As a person gets older, the body is less able to handle stress.

4. Discuss common disorders of the endocrine system

Matching

1. ____ Diabetes
2. ____ Diabetic peripheral neuropathy
3. ____ Diabetic retinopathy
4. ____ Goiter
5. ____ Hyperglycemia
6. ____ Hyperthyroidism
7. ____ Hypoglycemia
8. ____ Hypothyroidism
9. ____ Prediabetes
10. ____ Type 1 diabetes
11. ____ Type 2 diabetes

(A) Low blood glucose (blood sugar)

(B) High blood glucose (blood sugar)

(C) Condition in which the thyroid produces too much thyroid hormone, causing body processes to speed up

(D) Glucose levels are elevated but not high enough to establish diagnosis of diabetes

(E) Enlarged thyroid

(F) Condition in which the pancreas does not produce insulin or does not produce enough insulin

(G) Causes numbness, pain, or tingling of the legs and/or feet and nerve damage over time

(H) Causes damage to blood vessels in the eyes; can cause blindness

(I) Most common form and milder form of diabetes

(J) Condition in which the body lacks thyroid hormone, causing body processes to slow down

(K) Form of diabetes usually diagnosed in children and young adults

5. Describe care guidelines for diabetes

True or False

1. ____ If the nursing assistant notices any foot problems, such as a cut or sore on a resident's foot, she should wait approximately 24 hours before reporting it to see if it gets worse.

2. ____ Meals must be served at the same time every day for a resident who has diabetes.

3. ____ If a resident with diabetes is not following her diet, the nursing assistant should report it to the nurse.

4. ____ Blood glucose test strips should always be checked to make sure they have not expired.

5. ____ As long as a sore on a resident is small (dime-sized), it does not need to be reported.

6. ____ Nursing assistants should regularly trim a resident's toenails to help prevent complications of diabetes.

7. ____ Exercise is not recommended for people who have diabetes.

8. ____ Residents who have diabetes should go barefoot to improve circulation in their feet.

6. Discuss foot care guidelines for diabetes

Fill in the Blank

1. Diabetes weakens the _____ system, which reduces resistance to _____.

2. Poor _____ due to narrowing of the blood vessels increases the risk of infection.

3. When foot infections are not caught early, they can take months to heal. If wounds do not heal, _____ of a toe, foot, or leg may be necessary.

4. Foot care should be a part of _____ of residents and is required by CMS.

5. _____ soaps and _____ water should be avoided when bathing the feet.

6. The nursing assistant should not use any _____ to try to remove dirt from a toenail.

7. Using a doctor-recommended cream or lotion on the feet is fine, but nothing should be applied _____ the toes.

8. It is important for residents with diabetes not to walk around _____.

9. The nursing assistant should notify the nurse if a resident has excessively dry skin on the feet, breaks or tears in the skin, or a change in color of the skin or nails, especially _____ or _____.

24

The Immune and Lymphatic Systems and Cancer

1. Review the key terms in Learning Objective 1 before completing the workbook exercises

2. Explain the structure and function of the immune and lymphatic systems

Fill in the Blank

1. The immune system protects the body from disease-causing _____, viruses, and

   _____.

2. _____ immunity is present at birth; _____ immunity is acquired by the body.

3. In _____ immunity, the body manufactures antibodies as a response to a foreign substance; active immunity is also acquired by a

   _____.

4. With _____ immunity, a person is given the antibodies needed to defend against the antigen.

5. The lymphatic system is composed of lymph, lymph vessels, lymph

   _____, the spleen, and the _____ gland.

6. The clear yellowish fluid that moves into the lymph system and carries disease-fighting cells, lymphocytes, is called

   _____.

7. A main function of the spleen is to serve as a storage shed for _____.

3. Discuss changes in the immune and lymphatic systems due to aging

True or False

1. _____ Infections may increase with age.

2. _____ Vaccines are just as effective for older people as they are for younger people.

3. _____ Antibody response speeds up with age.

4. _____ T-cells decrease in number as a person gets older.

4. Describe a common disorder of the immune system

Short Answer

1. How does HIV harm the body?

   _____

   _____

   _____

   _____

   _____

2. List three common methods of HIV transmission.

   _____

   _____

   _____

   _____

   _____

   _____

3. List four common misconceptions about HIV transmission.

_____

_____

_____

_____

_____

_____

_____

_____

4. What is an opportunistic infection?

_____

_____

_____

_____

_____

_____

_____

5. A resident tells a nursing assistant that he accidentally touched another resident who has AIDS. He looks upset and says that he is very worried that he will now "catch it" himself. How should the nursing assistant respond?

_____

_____

_____

_____

_____

_____

_____

_____

_____

5. Discuss infection prevention guidelines for a resident with HIV/AIDS

Multiple Choice

1. Care for residents who have HIV or AIDS should focus on
   - (A) Helping to find a cure for HIV
   - (B) Preventing visits from friends and family
   - (C) Providing relief of symptoms and preventing infection
   - (D) Letting residents know what new medications are available to treat the disease

2. Confidentiality is especially important to people with HIV/AIDS because
   - (A) People with HIV/AIDS who are not working in health care can be fired from their jobs
   - (B) Others may pass judgment on people with this disease
   - (C) People can be forced to be tested for HIV
   - (D) Healthcare workers with HIV/AIDS can be fined if they do not disclose their illness

3. Which of the following is a guideline for preventing infection in residents with HIV?
   - (A) Personal items should not be shared.
   - (B) Sharps should be recapped carefully.
   - (C) Nursing assistants should wear masks when talking to the residents.
   - (D) Residents should be isolated from all other residents and most staff members.

6. Discuss care guidelines for a resident with HIV/AIDS

Multiple Choice

1. If a resident with AIDS has a poor appetite and is losing weight, the nursing assistant should
   - (A) Give him an over-the-counter appetite stimulant
   - (B) Report to the nurse if he is not eating or not enjoying his food
   - (C) Let the resident know that if he does not eat, he might die
   - (D) Discuss this with the resident's friends and family and see what they recommend doing

2. Which of the following statements is true of special diets for a resident who has AIDS?
(A) The resident will need to eat spicy foods.
(B) The resident will need to eat foods that are low in acid.
(C) The resident will need to eat high-fiber foods.
(D) The resident will need to eat very hot foods.

3. Someone who has nausea and vomiting may need to
(A) Eat mostly dairy products
(B) Eat small meals throughout the day
(C) Eat one large meal at bedtime
(D) Reduce liquid intake

4. The BRAT diet is helpful for
(A) Diarrhea
(B) Weight gain
(C) Nausea and vomiting
(D) Headaches

5. Fluids are important for residents who have diarrhea because
(A) Diarrhea causes the body to lose fluid
(B) Diarrhea can be prevented by drinking a lot of fluids
(C) Fluid intake is not important for a person who has diarrhea
(D) The nursing assistant will not have to offer the bedpan as often

7. Describe cancer

Matching

1. ____ Benign
2. ____ Biopsy
3. ____ Cancer
4. ____ Chemotherapy
5. ____ Hormone therapy
6. ____ Immunotherapy
7. ____ Malignant
8. ____ Metastasize
9. ____ Oncology
10. ____ Palliative care
11. ____ Radiation therapy
12. ____ Remission
13. ____ Surgery
14. ____ Tumor

(A) Noncancerous
(B) A group of abnormally growing cells
(C) To spread from the site where it first appeared to other areas of the body
(D) Cancerous
(E) Type of care that works to relieve symptoms and reduce pain and suffering
(F) Disappearance of signs and symptoms of cancer
(G) Can be effective when tumors rely on specific hormones to survive and grow
(H) Removal of a sample of tissue for examination and diagnosis
(I) Cancer vaccines are one form of this
(J) General term used to describe a disease in which abnormal cells grow in an uncontrolled way
(K) Uses high-energy rays to attempt to destroy cancer cells in a specific area
(L) Branch of medicine that deals with study and treatment of cancer
(M) Goal is to remove as much of the cancer as possible
(N) Chemical agents or medications are administered intravenously to kill malignant cells and tissues

8. Discuss care guidelines for a resident with cancer

Short Answer

For each of the following concerns for a resident with cancer, write one reason why it is important.

1. Preventing infection

_____

_____

_____

_____

2. Skin care

_____

_____

_____

_____

3. Mouth care

_____

_____

_____

_____

4. Nutrition

_____

_____

_____

_____

5. Bladder and bowel changes

_____

_____

_____

6. Mobility

_____

_____

_____

_____

7. Pain

_____

_____

_____

_____

8. Vital signs

_____

_____

_____

_____

9. Self-image

_____

_____

_____

_____

10. Mental status and emotional needs

_____

_____

_____

25

Rehabilitation and Restorative Care

1. Review the key terms in Learning Objective 1 before completing the workbook exercises

2. Discuss rehabilitation and restorative care

Short Answer

1. Define *rehabilitation*.

_____
_____
_____
_____
_____

2. List three goals of rehabilitative care.

_____
_____
_____
_____
_____
_____
_____

3. What do restorative care programs help with?

_____
_____
_____
_____
_____
_____
_____
_____

3. Describe the importance of promoting independence

True or False

1. ____ Being able to perform activities of daily living by oneself is not very important.

2. ____ Dressing is one example of an activity of daily living.

3. ____ Being required to accept help with activities of daily living can cause a decrease in independence.

4. ____ If a resident is doing a task too slowly, a nursing assistant should offer to do it for her to help prevent the resident from being frustrated.

5. ____ Independence helps with self-esteem and can help speed recovery.

6. ____ Verbal cues are short sequences of words that direct a person to complete a specific step.

7. ____ Residents have a legal right to make choices about food, visitors, and how to spend their time.

4. Explain the complications of immobility and describe how exercise helps maintain health

Short Answer
For each of these body systems, write one benefit of regular activity.

1. Gastrointestinal system:

_____

_____

2. Urinary system:

_____

_____

3. Integumentary system:

_____

_____

4. Circulatory system:

_____

_____

5. Respiratory system:

_____

_____

6. Musculoskeletal system:

_____

_____

7. Nervous system:

_____

_____

8. Endocrine system:

_____

_____

5. Describe canes, walkers, and crutches

Multiple Choice

1. How should a walker be moved?
   (A) Walker first, stronger leg, then weaker leg
   (B) Weaker leg, stronger leg, then walker
   (C) Stronger leg, walker, then weaker leg
   (D) Walker, weaker leg, then stronger leg

2. How many feet does a quad cane have?
   (A) Four
   (B) Three
   (C) Two
   (D) One

3. Which of the following walking aids is used when a resident cannot bear any weight at all on one leg?
   (A) C-cane
   (B) Quad cane
   (C) Walker
   (D) Crutches

4. Which of the following is true of using canes, walkers, and crutches?
   (A) A cane should be held on the resident's weaker side.
   (B) The resident should be wearing nonskid shoes with the laces tied.
   (C) When the resident is ambulating, the nursing assistant should stay near the resident's stronger side.
   (D) When the resident is ambulating, the nursing assistant should walk in front of the resident.

6. Discuss other assistive devices and orthotics

Fill in the Blank

1. _____ devices can help people who are recovering from illness or adapting to a physical disability.

2. _____ is a weakness of muscles in the feet and ankles that interferes with the ability to walk normally.

3. _____
   pillows or hip wedges keep hips in proper
   position after hip surgery.

4. Trochanter rolls prevent the hip and leg
   from turning _____.

5. Handrolls help prevent finger, hand, or wrist
   _____.

6. Orthotic devices are devices applied external-
   ly to a limb for _____
   and _____.

7. Discuss range of motion exercises

Matching
Use each letter only once.

1. _____ Abduction

2. _____ Active assisted range of motion
   (AAROM)

3. _____ Active range of motion (AROM)

4. _____ Adduction

5. _____ Dorsiflexion

6. _____ Extension

7. _____ Flexion

8. _____ Opposition

9. _____ Passive range of motion (PROM)

10. _____ Pronation

11. _____ Range of motion (ROM) exercises

12. _____ Rotation

13. _____ Supination

(A) Exercises done by a resident with some help
   from a staff member

(B) Straightening a body part

(C) Exercises that put a joint through its full arc
   of motion

(D) Turning downward

(E) Moving a body part away from the midline
   of the body

(F) Exercises done by a staff member, without
   the resident's help

(G) Turning upward

(H) Exercises done by a resident alone, without
   help

(I) Touching the thumb to any other finger

(J) Moving a body part toward the midline of
   the body

(K) Bending backward

(L) Bending a body part

(M) Turning the joint

Labeling
*In each of the blanks provided on the next page,
write the name of the range of motion body movement that is shown in the illustration.*

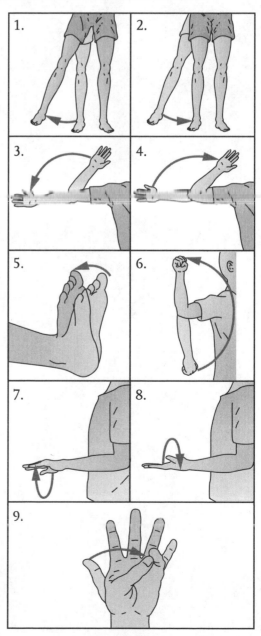

Name: _____

1. _____
2. _____
3. _____
4. _____
5. _____
6. _____
7. _____
8. _____
9. _____

26
Subacute Care

1. Review the key terms in Learning Objective 1 before completing the workbook exercises

2. Discuss the types of residents who are in a subacute setting

Short Answer

1. What is subacute care, and where is it usually provided?

_____

_____

_____

_____

_____

_____

_____

_____

2. List three conditions that might require subacute care.

_____

_____

_____

_____

_____

_____

_____

3. Describe preoperative and postoperative care

Multiple Choice

1. After having surgery that requires general anesthesia, the resident is usually moved to a(n)
    (A) Negative air pressure room
    (B) Postanesthesia care unit
    (C) Admitting and receiving area
    (D) Telemetry station

2. The medical abbreviation for a fluid restriction that means the resident cannot have anything by mouth is
    (A) OOB
    (B) MDR
    (C) CHF
    (D) NPO

3. A device that may need to be applied to prevent postoperative blood clots is a
    (A) Sterile bandage
    (B) Bath blanket
    (C) Sequential compression device
    (D) Fiberglass cast

4. How can an NA help a resident who is frightened or anxious before surgery?
    (A) By being compassionate and listening
    (B) By telling the resident about nonsurgical methods she can try first
    (C) By letting the resident know she is worrying too much
    (D) By discussing the resident's postoperative medical orders

Name: _____

4. List care guidelines for pulse oximetry

True or False

1. _____ A pulse oximeter measures a person's blood oxygen level and pulse rate.

2. _____ A normal blood oxygen level is approximately 84%.

3. _____ Diseases such as chronic obstructive pulmonary disease can lower a person's blood oxygen level.

4. _____ If the alarm on the pulse oximeter sounds, the nursing assistant should turn it off.

5. _____ The nursing assistant should report cyanotic skin or mucous membranes.

5. Describe telemetry and list care guidelines

Fill in the Blank

1. Telemetry is the application of a

_____

monitoring device.

2. The telemetry unit transmits information about the heart's _____

and _____

to a central monitoring station.

3. A portable telemetry unit attaches to a resident's _____.

4. The nursing assistant should monitor _____ carefully

as ordered.

5. The nursing assistant should report if electrodes become _____.

6. Explain artificial airways and list care guidelines

Multiple Choice

1. An artificial airway may be needed in order to facilitate
   (A) Ventilation
   (B) Secretions
   (C) Heart rate
   (D) Aspiration

2. An opening through the neck into the trachea is called a(n)
   (A) Ileostomy
   (B) Gastrostomy
   (C) Colostomy
   (D) Tracheostomy

3. When assisting a resident with an artificial airway, the nursing assistant should
   (A) Avoid performing mouth care on the resident so that the airway does not become blocked
   (B) Use other methods of communication, such as writing notes or communication boards, if the resident cannot speak
   (C) Reinsert the tubing if it falls out
   (D) Give medication to relax the resident if he bites or tugs on the tube

7. Discuss care for a resident with a tracheostomy

Crossword Puzzle

Across

3. A nursing assistant should provide this for the site around the tracheostomy

4. One position that a resident may need to be in when he has a tracheostomy

5. A cuffless tracheostomy tube is often used if the resident has a low risk for this

Down

1. One reason why a tracheostomy may be necessary

2. A person with a tracheostomy may not be able to do this

3. Another name for the opening for the tracheostomy

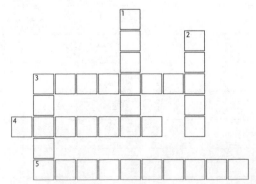

8. Describe mechanical ventilation and explain care guidelines

True or False

1. ____ A ventilator performs the process of breathing for a person who cannot breathe on his own.

2. ____ A resident using a mechanical ventilator is usually able to speak, although his voice will be weaker.

3. ____ A resident using a mechanical ventilator will prefer to be left alone as much as possible.

4. ____ A resident using a mechanical ventilator is often sedated.

5. ____ A resident using a mechanical ventilator needs to be positioned flat on his back at all times.

6. ____ The nursing assistant should reposition a resident using a mechanical ventilator at least every two hours.

7. ____ Residents using mechanical ventilators will require one-on-one care during a power failure.

8. ____ Most residents using mechanical ventilators will show nervousness or anxiety, so it is not necessary for the nursing assistant to notify the nurse if this occurs.

9. Describe suctioning and list signs of respiratory distress

Short Answer

1. When is suctioning needed?

2. List four signs of respiratory distress.

3. List six guidelines for suctioning.

10. Describe chest tubes and explain related care

Multiple Choice

1. Chest tubes are inserted during a _____ procedure.
   (A) Sterile
   (B) Nonsterile
   (C) Nasogastric
   (D) Catheterized

Name: _____

2. Chest tubes drain air, blood, or fluid from
    (A) The heart
    (B) The brain
    (C) The pleural cavity
    (D) The esophagus

3. Chest tubes may be required for
    (A) Vaginitis
    (B) Eczema
    (C) Nutritional deficiencies
    (D) Surgery or injuries

4. The drainage system for the chest tube must be
    (A) Recycled
    (B) Permanent
    (C) Airtight
    (D) Frozen

5. The drainage system for the chest tube must be kept _____ the level of the resident's chest.
    (A) Above
    (B) Below
    (C) Beside
    (D) At the same height as

11. Describe alternative feeding methods and related care

Matching
Use each letter only once.

1. _____ Central venous line

2. _____ Gastric suctioning

3. _____ Gastrostomy

4. _____ Nasogastric tube

5. _____ Percutaneous endoscopic gastrostomy (PEG) tube

6. _____ Total parenteral nutrition (TPN)

(A) Tube placed through the abdominal wall into the stomach

(B) Tube inserted into the nose, down the back of the throat through the esophagus, and into the stomach

(C) Nutrients are received intravenously, bypassing the digestive tract

(D) Surgically created opening in the abdomen and the stomach through which a PEG tube is placed

(E) Placed in one of the larger veins in the body when total parenteral nutrition is expected to be continued for a period of time

(F) May be used postoperatively for the removal of materials inside the body via suctioning

12. Discuss care guidelines for dialysis

Short Answer

1. What is kidney dialysis and why is it used?

_____
_____
_____
_____
_____
_____
_____

2. List five things that a nursing assistant should report to the nurse about dialysis.

_____
_____
_____
_____
_____
_____
_____
_____
_____
_____
_____
_____
_____

27

End-of-Life Care

1. Review the key terms in Learning Objective 1 before completing the workbook exercises

2. Describe palliative care

Short Answer

1. When is palliative care given?

_____
_____
_____
_____
_____
_____
_____

2. List four goals of palliative care.

_____
_____
_____
_____
_____
_____
_____
_____
_____
_____
_____

3. Discuss hospice care

True or False

1. ____ Hospice care is ordered by a doctor when a person has approximately six months or less to live.

2. ____ Hospice care is generally not available on Sundays.

3. ____ Hospice care focuses on curing the person's disease or disorder.

4. ____ Hospice care focuses on making residents comfortable and managing their pain.

5. ____ Hospice care uses a holistic approach.

6. ____ The resident's family is not involved in hospice care.

4. Discuss the grief process and related terms

Multiple Choice

1. Mr. Anderson, a resident, talks to God about his terminal cancer. He promises to make peace with his estranged son if he is allowed to live. Which stage of dying is Mr. Anderson going through?
    (A) Denial
    (B) Anger
    (C) Bargaining
    (D) Depression
    (E) Acceptance

End-of-Life Care

2. Russell, a nursing assistant, knows that his resident, Ms. Wilson, is dying. One day Ms. Wilson begins to yell at Russell, blaming him for a lack of proper care, saying, "If you had been a better caregiver, I would never have gotten sick." Russell tries to comfort her, not taking it personally because he realizes that this is the _____ stage of dying.
(A) Denial
(B) Anger
(C) Bargaining
(D) Depression
(E) Acceptance

3. Mrs. Curry is a resident who is dying. She has an appointment with her attorney. When he visits her in her room, he says, "I just want to make sure everything is in order with your will." She thanks him nicely but tells him she has no idea why he would want to talk about that subject. Instead she wants to talk about her son. Which stage of dying is Mrs. Curry in?
(A) Denial
(B) Anger
(C) Bargaining
(D) Depression
(E) Acceptance

4. Gwen, a nursing assistant, notices that her resident, Wes, seems a little distant. When he talks to her, he only wants to discuss the specifics of his funeral arrangements. He is very concerned about making sure his family is taken care of after he is gone. Gwen takes notes on everything he says. In which stage of dying is Wes?
(A) Denial
(B) Anger
(C) Bargaining
(D) Depression
(E) Acceptance

5. Angelica, a nursing assistant, is worried about one of her terminally ill residents. He alternates between crying and not talking to anyone. This resident is experiencing _____.
(A) Denial
(B) Anger
(C) Bargaining
(D) Depression
(E) Acceptance

5. Explain legal rights for a resident who is dying

Short Answer
For each of the rights of a dying person listed below, write one way that a nursing assistant can honor that right.

1. The right to have visitors

_____

_____

_____

_____

2. The right to privacy

_____

_____

_____

_____

3. The right to be free from pain

_____

_____

_____

_____

4. The right to honest and accurate information

_____

_____

_____

_____

5. The right to refuse treatment

_____

_____

_____

_____

6. Explain how to care for a resident who is dying

Short Answer

Make a check mark (✓) by each suggestion below that describes a helpful way for a nursing assistant to care for a resident who is dying.

1. _____ Use alternative methods of communication if speech fails.

2. _____ Stop talking because the resident is probably unaware of his surroundings.

3. _____ Keep the room softly lit.

4. _____ Turn and position the resident often.

5. _____ Change gowns and sheets regularly.

6. _____ Feed the resident quickly.

7. _____ Observe resident for signs of pain.

8. _____ Insist that the resident eat and drink because it will prolong his life.

9. _____ Clean the resident immediately after episodes of incontinence.

7. Discuss factors that influence feelings about death and list ways to meet residents' individual needs

Short Answer

1. Briefly describe some ideas about death that are part of your cultural beliefs or another culture that you are familiar with.

_____

_____

_____

_____

_____

_____

_____

_____

_____

2. Have you ever experienced the death of a loved one? If so, how did you grieve?

_____

_____

_____

_____

_____

_____

_____

_____

_____

_____

3. Why do you think the text states, "Listen more; talk less"?

_____

_____

_____

_____

_____

_____

_____

_____

_____

_____

_____

_____

Name: _____

8. Identify common signs of approaching death

Fill in the Blank

Make a check mark (✓) beside the signs of approaching death.

1. ____ High blood pressure

2. ____ Fever

3. ____ Cold, pale skin

4. ____ Confusion

5. ____ Healthy skin tone

6. ____ Heightened sense of touch

7. ____ Inability to speak

8. ____ Incontinence

9. ____ Perspiration

10. ____ Normal, quiet breathing

9. List changes that may occur in the human body after death

Fill in the Blank

1. When death occurs, the body will not have a pulse, respiration, or

   _____.

2. The _____ drops, causing the mouth to stay

   _____.

3. _____ may be partially open with eyes in a

   _____.

4. Resident may have both

   _____ and

   _____

   incontinence.

5. The pupils will be

   _____ and

   _____.

10. Describe ways to help family and friends deal with a resident's death

True or False

1. ____ If a family member becomes very upset after a loved one's death, it is helpful for the nursing assistant to ask him to calm down and to stop crying.

2. ____ Family and friends may feel guilt after a loved one's death, especially if there were unresolved issues in the relationship.

3. ____ If family members seem relieved after a loved one has died, it means that they did not care for the resident very much.

4. ____ A nursing assistant should let family members and friends talk about their feelings without interrupting them.

5. ____ A nursing assistant should not let a resident's friends know that she is upset about the resident's death.

6. ____ Reassuring family and friends that they will get over the death of their loved one is helpful.

11. Describe ways to help staff members cope with a resident's death

Short Answer

1. If a nursing assistant wants to attend a resident's memorial service that is being held at a funeral home, what should she do first?

   _____

   _____

   _____

   _____

   _____

2. List five ways that staff members can cope with the death of a resident.

_____

_____

_____

_____

_____

_____

12. Describe postmortem care

Multiple Choice

1. Which of the following terms means care of the body after death?
    (A) Hospice care
    (B) Postmortem care
    (C) Palliative care
    (D) Fixed care

2. What is the purpose of an autopsy?
    (A) To determine how to dispose of the resident's belongings
    (B) To determine the cause of death
    (C) To determine where the resident wants to be buried
    (D) To determine if the resident wants to be an organ donor

3. Generally speaking, how should a nursing assistant position a resident's body after the resident has died?
    (A) The resident should be placed on her back.
    (B) The resident should be placed on her side.
    (C) The resident should be placed on her abdomen.
    (D) The resident should be placed sitting as upright as possible.

4. Where are drainage pads most often needed after a person has died?
    (A) Under the arms
    (B) Under the feet
    (C) Under the perineal area
    (D) Under the calves

Name: _____

28

Your New Position

1. Review the key terms in Learning Objective 1 before completing the workbook exercises

2. Describe how to write a résumé and cover letter

True or False

1. ____ A person should explain his entire work history in his cover letter.

2. ____ It is best that a person's education not be listed on his résumé.

3. ____ The first step in any job search is to prepare a résumé.

4. ____ A résumé should be approximately three pages long.

5. ____ A cover letter should include information on why the person is seeking the job and why he is qualified for the position.

3. Identify information that may be required for filling out a job application

Short Answer
Complete the sample job application.

Employment Application

Personal Information

Name:	Date:

Home Address:

City, State, Zip:

Email Address:

Home Phone:	Business Phone:

US Citizen?	If Not, Give Visa No. and Expiration Date:

Position Applying For

Title:	Salary Desired:

Referred By:	Date Available:

Education

High School (Name, City, State):

Graduation Date:

Technical or Undergraduate School:

Dates Attended:	Degree Major:

References

4. Discuss proper grooming guidelines for a job interview

Short Answer

Make a check mark (✓) next to the descriptions that are appropriate for job interviews.

1. ____ Wearing rings on every finger

2. ____ Brushing teeth beforehand

3. ____ Smoking a cigarette right before the interview to calm down

4. ____ Not wearing perfume or cologne

5. ____ Wearing jeans

6. ____ Wearing high-heeled black sandals

7. ____ Wearing artificial, painted nails

8. ____ Not wearing shorts

5. List techniques for interviewing successfully

Short Answer

Make a check mark (✓) next to the behaviors that are appropriate for job interviews.

1. ____ Looking around the room while you are being interviewed

2. ____ Shaking hands firmly with the interviewer

3. ____ Practicing for the interview

4. ____ Not smiling during the interview

5. ____ Arriving 10 to 15 minutes early for the interview

6. ____ Exaggerating accomplishments to sound more appealing

7. ____ Sending a follow-up thank-you note

6. Describe a standard job description and list steps for following the scope of practice

Crossword Puzzle

Across

3. What a nursing assistant must do with a job description before signing it

4. An outline of what will be expected in a job

Down

1. If this is not listed in a job description, it should not be performed

2. If a nursing assistant has forgotten how to perform a procedure, she should ask this professional for a reminder

5. Possible result to resident, another staff member, or NA when an NA does something outside of her scope of practice

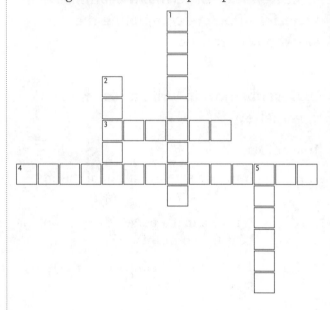

7. Identify guidelines for maintaining certification and explain the state's registry

Multiple Choice

1. According to OBRA, what is the minimum number of hours of training a nursing assistant must complete before being employed?
   (A) 50
   (B) 64
   (C) 75
   (D) 110

2. Within how many months of training must a nursing assistant usually take the state test?
   (A) Six months
   (B) 12 months
   (C) 18 months
   (D) 24 months

3. In most states, a nursing assistant has _____ chance(s) to pass the state test.
   (A) One
   (B) Two
   (C) Three
   (D) Four

4. Which of the following is an example of information kept in the state registry for nursing assistants?
   (A) Information about investigations regarding abuse, neglect, or theft
   (B) The nursing assistant's medical records
   (C) The resident's medical records
   (D) The nursing assistant's family's medical records

8. Describe continuing education for nursing assistants

True or False

1. _____ OBRA requires that nursing assistants must have 12 hours of continuing education each year in order to keep certification current.

2. _____ The continuing education requirement for all states is the same as OBRA's.

3. _____ Subjects covered in continuing education include Residents' Rights, infection prevention, and confidentiality.

4. _____ Employers are required to provide free hepatitis B vaccines for all employees.

9. Describe employee evaluations and discuss feedback

Fill in the Blank

1. An annual _____, sometimes called a performance _____ or review, is used to evaluate the performance of each employee.

2. Employees may be evaluated on overall _____, _____ resolution, and _____ effort.

3. _____ feedback involves giving opinions about the work of others, which includes helpful suggestions for change.

4. _____ criticism is angry and negative and should not be given in the workplace.

5. When receiving constructive feedback, the nursing assistant should be _____ to suggestions.

6. If a nursing assistant is not sure how to avoid a _____ he has made, he should ask for suggestions.

7. Performance reviews are frequently the basis for _____.

8. A satisfactory review can increase chances of _____ within the facility.

10. Discuss conflict resolution

Short Answer

1. What is conflict resolution?

   _____
   _____
   _____
   _____
   _____
   _____
   _____
   _____

2. What should a nursing assistant always do when changing jobs?

   _____
   _____
   _____
   _____

Name: _____

11. Define *stress* and explain ways to manage stress

Matching
Use each letter only once.

1. _____ Abdominal breathing

2. _____ Burnout

3. _____ Increasing exercise, developing new hobbies, setting realistic goals

4. _____ Residents and residents' families

5. _____ Smoking, increasing caffeine in the diet, taking illegal drugs

6. _____ Stress

7. _____ Stressor

8. _____ Supervisor, doctor, friends and family, spiritual leader

(A) An internal or external factor or stimulus that causes stress

(B) Mental or physical exhaustion due to a prolonged period of stress and frustration

(C) Unhealthy responses to stress

(D) A relaxation technique for managing stress

(E) Appropriate people to turn to for help with stress

(F) Healthy ways to manage stress

(G) Inappropriate people to talk to about stress

(H) Mentally or emotionally disruptive or upsetting condition that occurs due to changes in the environment

12. Describe how to be a valued member of the healthcare community

Short Answer

1. List two people to thank for helping you to complete your nursing assistant training course.

_____

_____

_____

2. Describe one thing you are going to do to reward yourself for meeting this goal.

_____

_____

_____

_____

_____

_____

3. List one thing you will do to keep learning as you move forward in your new profession.

_____

_____

_____

_____

_____

_____

Procedure Checklists

6
Infection Prevention and Control

Washing hands (hand hygiene)			
		yes	no
1.	Turns on water at the sink. Keeps clothes dry and does not let clothing touch the outside portion of the sink or counter.		
2.	Wets hands and wrists thoroughly.		
3.	Applies soap to hands.		
4.	Keeps hands lower than elbows and fingertips down. Rubs hands together and fingers between each other to create a lather. Lathers all surfaces of wrists, fingers, and hands, using friction for at least 20 seconds.		
5.	Cleans nails by rubbing them in the palm of other hand.		
6.	Keeps hands lower than elbows and fingertips down. Rinses thoroughly under running water. Rinses all surfaces of wrists, hands, and fingers. Runs water down from wrists to fingertips.		
7.	Uses a clean, dry paper towel to dry all surfaces of fingers, hands, and wrists. Discards towel without touching waste container.		
8.	Uses clean, dry paper towel to turn off the faucet. Discards paper towel into waste container. Does not contaminate hands by touching the surface of the sink or faucet.		

_____   _____
Date Reviewed   Instructor Signature

_____   _____
Date Performed   Instructor Signature

Putting on (donning) gloves			
		yes	no
1.	Washes hands.		
2.	If right-handed, slides one glove on left hand (reverses if left-handed).		
3.	Using gloved hand, slides the other hand into the second glove.		
4.	Interlaces fingers to smooth out folds and create a comfortable fit.		
5.	Checks for tears, holes, cracks, or discolored spots. Replaces the glove if needed.		
6.	Adjusts gloves until they are pulled up over the wrists and fit correctly. If wearing a gown, pulls cuffs of the gloves over the sleeves of the gown.		

_____   _____
Date Reviewed   Instructor Signature

_____   _____
Date Performed   Instructor Signature

Removing (doffing) gloves			
		yes	no
1.	Touching only the outside of one glove with one gloved hand, grasps the other glove at the palm and pulls the glove off.		
2.	With the fingertips of gloved hand, holds glove just removed. With ungloved hand, slips two fingers underneath cuff of the remaining glove at wrist. Does not touch any part of the outside of the glove.		
3.	Pulls down, turning this glove inside out and over the first glove as it is removed.		

Name: _____

		yes	no
4.	One glove is now held from its clean inner side. The other glove is inside it.		
5.	Drops both gloves into the proper container without contaminating self.		
6.	Washes hands.		

_____   _____
Date Reviewed   Instructor Signature

_____   _____
Date Performed   Instructor Signature

Putting on (donning) and removing (doffing) gown

		yes	no
1.	Washes hands.		
2.	Opens the gown. Holds it out in front of self and allows it to open/unfold. Does not shake gown or touch it to the floor. Facing the back opening of the gown, places arms through each sleeve.		
3.	Fastens neck opening.		
4.	Reaches behind self and pulls gown until it completely covers clothing. Secures gown at waist.		
5.	When removing gown, removes and discards gloves first. Unfastens gown at neck and waist and does not touch the outside of gown. Holds gown away from body and rolls dirty side in. Discards gown in proper container. Avoids touching any surface in the room.		

_____   _____
Date Reviewed   Instructor Signature

_____   _____
Date Performed   Instructor Signature

Putting on (donning) mask and goggles

		yes	no
1.	Washes hands.		
2.	Picks up the mask by the top strings or the elastic strap. Does not touch the mask where it touches face.		
3.	Pulls strap over head or ties top strings, then bottom strings.		
4.	Pinches metal strip at the top of the mask tightly around nose so that it feels snug. Fits mask snugly around face and below the chin.		
5.	Puts on goggles over the eyes or eyeglasses. Secures them to the head using the headband or earpieces.		
6.	Puts on gloves after putting on mask and goggles.		

_____   _____
Date Reviewed   Instructor Signature

_____   _____
Date Performed   Instructor Signature

Donning and doffing a full set of PPE

		yes	no
	Donning:		
1.	Washes hands.		
2.	Puts on gown.		
3.	Puts on mask or respirator.		
4.	Puts on goggles or face shield.		
5.	Puts on gloves.		
	Doffing:		
1.	Removes and discards gloves.		
2.	Removes goggles or face shield.		
3.	Removes and discards gown.		
4.	Removes and discards mask.		
5.	Washes hands.		

_____   _____
Date Reviewed   Instructor Signature

_____   _____
Date Performed   Instructor Signature

8
Emergency Care, First Aid, and Disasters

Performing abdominal thrusts for the conscious person

		yes	no
1.	Stands behind the person. Brings arms under person's arms. Wraps arms around person's waist.		
2.	Makes a fist with one hand. Places flat, thumb side of the fist against person's abdomen, above the navel but below the breastbone.		
3.	Grasps fist with other hand. Pulls both hands toward self and up (inward and upward), quickly and forcefully.		
4.	Repeats until the object is pushed out.		

Date Reviewed _____ Instructor Signature _____

Date Performed _____ Instructor Signature _____

Responding to shock

		yes	no
1.	Notifies nurse immediately.		
2.	If controlling bleeding, puts on gloves first.		
3.	Has person lie down on her back. Elevates legs.		
4.	Checks pulse and respirations; begins CPR if breathing and pulse are absent and if trained.		
5.	Keeps person as calm and comfortable as possible. Loosens clothing around neck and any belt/string around waist.		
6.	Maintains normal body temperature.		
7.	Does not give person food or liquids.		

Date Reviewed _____ Instructor Signature _____

Date Performed _____ Instructor Signature _____

Controlling bleeding

		yes	no
1.	Notifies nurse immediately.		
2.	Puts on gloves.		
3.	Holds thick sterile pad, clean cloth, or clean towel against the wound.		
4.	Presses down hard directly on the bleeding wound until help arrives. Does not decrease pressure. Puts additional pads over first pad if blood seeps through. Does not remove first pad.		
5.	Raises wound above level of the heart to slow down bleeding. Props up limb.		
6.	When bleeding is under control, secures dressing to keep it in place. Checks person for symptoms of shock. Stays with person until help arrives.		
7.	Removes and discards gloves and washes hands thoroughly.		

Date Reviewed _____ Instructor Signature _____

Date Performed _____ Instructor Signature _____

Treating burns

		yes	no
	To treat a minor burn:		
1.	Notifies nurse immediately. Puts on gloves.		

2.	Uses cool, clean water to decrease the skin temperature and prevent further injury. Does not use ice or ice water. Dampens clean cloth with cool water, and places it over the burn.		
3.	Once the pain has eased, covers area with a dry, clean dressing or nonadhesive sterile bandage.		
4.	Removes and discards gloves. Washes hands.		
	For more serious burns:		
1.	Removes person from the source of the burn. If clothing has caught fire, has person stop, drop, and roll, or smothers the fire with a blanket or towel. Protects self from source of the burn.		
2.	Notifies nurse immediately. Puts on gloves.		
3.	Checks for breathing, pulse, and severe bleeding. If the person is not breathing and has no pulse, begins CPR if trained to do so. Does not put pillows under the head.		
4.	Does not use any type of ointment, water, salve, or grease on the burn.		
5.	Does not try to pull away any clothing from burned areas. Covers burn lightly with sterile gauze or a clean sheet. Does not rub the burned area.		
6.	Takes steps to prevent shock.		
7.	Does not give person food or liquids.		
8.	Monitors vital signs and waits for emergency medical help.		
9.	Removes and discards gloves. Washes hands.		

_____   _____
Date Reviewed   Instructor Signature

_____   _____
Date Performed   Instructor Signature

Responding to fainting

		yes	no
1.	Notifies nurse immediately.		
2.	Has person lie down or sit down before fainting occurs.		
3.	If person is in a sitting position, has him bend forward and place his head between his knees. If the person is lying flat on his back, elevates the legs.		
4.	Loosens any tight clothing.		
5.	Has person stay in this position for at least five minutes after symptoms disappear.		
6.	Helps person get up slowly. Continues to observe him for symptoms of fainting. Uses call light if help is needed but person cannot be left alone.		
7.	If person faints, lowers him to floor, positioning him on his back. Keeps him lying down for several minutes and reports the incident.		

_____   _____
Date Reviewed   Instructor Signature

_____   _____
Date Performed   Instructor Signature

Responding to a nosebleed

		yes	no
1.	Notifies nurse immediately.		
2.	Elevates head of the bed, or tells person to remain in a sitting position, leaning forward slightly. Offers tissues, a clean cloth, or emesis basin to catch the blood. Does not touch blood or bloody clothes, tissues, or cloths without gloves.		
3.	Puts on gloves. Applies firm pressure on both sides of the nose, on the soft part near the bridge. Squeezes sides with thumb and forefinger.		

4.	Applies pressure until the bleeding stops.		
5.	Uses cool cloth or ice wrapped in a cloth over the bridge of the nose to slow the flow of blood. Does not apply ice directly to skin.		
6.	Keeps person still and calm until help arrives.		
7.	Removes and discards gloves. Washes hands.		

_____   _____
Date Reviewed   Instructor Signature

_____   _____
Date Performed   Instructor Signature

Responding to vomiting

		yes	no
1.	Notifies nurse immediately.		
2.	Puts on gloves.		
3.	Places an emesis basin under the chin. Removes basin when vomiting has stopped		
4.	Removes used linens or clothes. Replaces with fresh linens or clothes.		
5.	Notes amount, color, and consistency of vomitus. Looks for blood in vomitus, blood-tinged vomitus, or medication (pills) in vomitus. Shows nurse the vomitus before discarding if blood or pills are noted.		
6.	Flushes vomitus down the toilet and washes and stores basin.		
7.	Removes and discards gloves.		
8.	Washes hands.		
9.	Puts on fresh gloves.		
10.	Provides comfort to the person. Provides mouth care.		
11.	Puts used linen in proper containers.		
12.	Removes and discards gloves.		

13.	Washes hands again.		
14.	Documents time, amount, color, odor, and consistency of vomitus.		

_____   _____
Date Reviewed   Instructor Signature

_____   _____
Date Performed   Instructor Signature

Responding to a myocardial infarction

		yes	no
1.	Notifies nurse immediately.		
2.	Places the person in a comfortable position. Encourages him to rest. Reassures person that he will not be left alone.		
3.	Loosens clothing around the person's neck.		
4.	Does not give person food or liquids.		
5.	Monitors person's breathing and pulse. If person is not breathing and has no pulse, begins CPR if trained.		
6.	Stays with person until help has arrived.		

_____   _____
Date Reviewed   Instructor Signature

_____   _____
Date Performed   Instructor Signature

Responding to seizures

		yes	no
1.	Notes the time. Puts on gloves. Removes person's eyeglasses.		
2.	Lowers person to the floor. Cradles and protects his head. Loosens clothing to help with breathing. Attempts to turn his head to one side to lower the risk of choking.		
3.	Has someone call the nurse immediately or uses call light. Does not leave person.		
4.	Moves furniture away.		

		yes	no
5.	Does not try to stop the seizure or restrain person.		
6.	Does not force anything between person's teeth. Does not place hands in his mouth for any reason.		
7.	Does not give person food or liquids.		
8.	When the seizure is over, notes the time. Gently turns person to his left side. Checks for adequate breathing and pulse. If the person is not breathing and has no pulse, begins CPR if trained.		
9.	Removes and discards gloves. Washes hands.		
10.	Reports length of the seizure and observations to the nurse.		

_____   _____
Date Reviewed   Instructor Signature

_____   _____
Date Performed   Instructor Signature

9
Admission, Transfer, Discharge, and Physical Exams

Admitting a resident			
		yes	no
1.	Identifies self by name. Identifies resident. Greets resident by name.		
2.	Washes hands.		
3.	Explains procedure to resident. Speaks clearly, slowly, and directly. Maintains face-to-face contact whenever possible.		
4.	Provides for resident's privacy with a curtain, screen, or door. Shows family where to wait.		
5.	If instructed, does these things:		
	Measures resident's height, weight, and vital signs. Documents on admission form and elsewhere per facility policy.		

		yes	no
	Obtains a urine specimen if required.		
	Completes the paperwork. Takes an inventory of all the personal items. Helps resident put personal items away. Labels each item if facility policy. If resident has valuables, asks nurse for instructions.		
	Fills the water pitcher with fresh water. Adds ice if requested.		
6.	Locates family and lets them know they may return to resident's room.		
7.	Shows resident the room and bathroom. Explains how to work bed controls and call light. Points out the lights, telephone, and television and how to work them. Gives resident information on menus, dining times, and activity schedules.		
8.	Introduces resident to his roommate if there is one. Introduces other residents and staff.		
9.	Makes resident comfortable. Removes privacy measures.		
10.	Leaves call light within resident's reach.		
11.	Washes hands.		
12.	Is courteous and respectful at all times. Asks resident if he needs anything else.		
13.	Documents procedure using facility guidelines.		

_____   _____
Date Reviewed   Instructor Signature

_____   _____
Date Performed   Instructor Signature

Measuring and recording weight of an ambulatory resident			
		yes	no
1.	Identifies self by name. Identifies resident. Greets resident by name.		
2.	Washes hands.		

3.	Explains procedure to resident. Speaks clearly, slowly, and directly. Maintains face-to-face contact whenever possible.		
4.	Provides for resident's privacy with a curtain, screen, or door.		
5.	Makes sure resident is wearing nonskid shoes before walking to scale.		
6.	Starts with the scale balanced at zero.		
7.	Helps resident step onto the center of the scale, facing the scale.		
8.	Determines resident's weight.		
9.	Helps resident off the scale before recording weight.		
10.	Removes privacy measures.		
11.	Leaves call light within resident's reach.		
12.	Washes hands.		
13.	Is courteous and respectful at all times.		
14.	Reports any changes in resident to the nurse. Records the resident's weight in pounds (lb) or kilograms (kg). Documents procedure using facility guidelines.		

_____   _____
Date Reviewed   Instructor Signature

_____   _____
Date Performed   Instructor Signature

Measuring and recording weight of a bedridden resident

		yes	no
1.	Identifies self by name. Identifies resident. Greets resident by name.		
2.	Washes hands.		
3.	Explains procedure to resident. Speaks clearly, slowly, and directly. Maintains face-to-face contact whenever possible.		
4.	Provides for resident's privacy with a curtain, screen, or door.		

5.	Adjusts bed to a safe level, usually waist high. Locks bed wheels.		
6.	Starts with scale balanced at zero.		
7.	Examines sling, straps, chains, and/or pad for any damage.		
8.	Turns linen down.		
9.	Turns resident toward self. Slides resident onto pad or sling.		
10.	Turns resident on his back and straightens sling.		
11.	Attaches sling to the scale or positions resident securely on the pad.		
12.	Checks straps or other connectors, and raises the sling or the pad until the resident is clear of the bed. Secures resident before moving the scale.		
13.	For digital scales, turns them on and notes reading. With other scales, moves weights until reading is apparent. Notes weight.		
14.	Lowers resident back down on the bed. Removes sling or slides resident back onto bed.		
15.	Makes resident comfortable. Replaces bed linens.		
16.	Returns bed to lowest position. Removes privacy measures.		
17.	Leaves call light within resident's reach.		
18.	Washes hands.		
19.	Is courteous and respectful at all times.		
20.	Reports any changes in resident to the nurse. Records the resident's weight in pounds (lb) or kilograms (kg). Documents procedure using facility guidelines.		

_____   _____
Date Reviewed   Instructor Signature

_____   _____
Date Performed   Instructor Signature

154

Name: _____

	Measuring and recording height of an ambulatory resident	yes	no
1.	Identifies self by name. Identifies resident. Greets resident by name.		
2.	Washes hands.		
3.	Explains procedure to resident. Speaks clearly, slowly, and directly. Maintains face-to-face contact whenever possible.		
4.	Provides for resident's privacy with a curtain, screen, or door.		
5.	Makes sure resident is wearing nonskid shoes before walking to scale.		
6.	Helps resident to step onto scale, facing away from the scale.		
7.	Asks resident to stand straight if possible. Helps as needed.		
8.	Pulls up measuring rod from back of scale. Lowers measuring rod until it rests flat on the resident's head.		
9.	Determines resident's height.		
10.	Helps resident off scale.		
11.	Removes privacy measures.		
12.	Leaves call light within resident's reach.		
13.	Washes hands.		
14.	Is courteous and respectful at all times.		
15.	Reports any changes in resident to the nurse. Records resident's height. Documents procedure using facility guidelines.		

_____ _____
Date Reviewed   Instructor Signature

_____ _____
Date Performed   Instructor Signature

	Measuring and recording height of a bedridden resident	yes	no
1.	Identifies self by name. Identifies resident. Greets resident by name.		
2.	Washes hands.		
3.	Explains procedure to resident. Speaks clearly, slowly, and directly. Maintains face-to-face contact whenever possible.		
4.	Provides for resident's privacy with a curtain, screen, or door.		
5.	Adjusts bed to a safe level, usually waist high. Locks bed wheels.		
6.	Turns linen down so it is off resident.		
7.	Positions resident lying straight in the supine (back) position.		
8.	Using a pencil, makes small mark on the bottom sheet at the top of the resident's head.		
9.	Makes another pencil mark at the resident's heel.		
10.	Using the tape measure, measures area between pencil marks.		
11.	Makes resident comfortable. Replaces bed linen.		
12.	Returns bed to lowest position. Removes privacy measures.		
13.	Leaves call light within resident's reach.		
14.	Washes hands.		
15.	Is courteous and respectful at all times.		
16.	Reports any changes in resident to the nurse. Records resident's height. Documents procedure using facility guidelines.		

_____ _____
Date Reviewed   Instructor Signature

_____ _____
Date Performed   Instructor Signature

Name: _____

Transferring a resident to a new room

		yes	no
1.	Identifies self by name. Identifies resident. Greets resident by name.		
2.	Washes hands.		
3.	Explains procedure to resident. Speaks clearly, slowly, and directly. Maintains face-to-face contact whenever possible.		
4.	Provides for resident's privacy with a curtain, screen, or door.		
5.	Collects items to be moved onto the cart, and asks another staff member to help take them to the new location.		
6.	Locks wheelchair or stretcher wheels. Helps resident into wheelchair or onto the stretcher. Takes him to the new area.		
7.	Introduces resident to new residents and staff.		
8.	Provides for resident's privacy with a curtain, screen, or door.		
9.	Locks wheelchair or stretcher wheels. Transfers resident to the new bed if needed.		
10.	Unpacks all belongings. Helps resident put personal items away.		
11.	Makes resident comfortable. Removes privacy measures.		
12.	Leaves call light within resident's reach.		
13.	Washes hands.		
14.	Is courteous and respectful at all times.		
15.	Reports to charge nurse. Reports any changes in resident to the nurse. Documents procedure using facility guidelines.		

_____ _____
Date Reviewed   Instructor Signature
_____ _____
Date Performed   Instructor Signature

Discharging a resident

		yes	no
1.	Identifies self by name. Identifies resident. Greets resident by name.		
2.	Washes hands.		
3.	Explains procedure to resident. Speaks clearly, slowly, and directly. Maintains face-to-face contact whenever possible.		
4.	Provides for resident's privacy with a curtain, screen, or door.		
5.	Measures vital signs.		
6.	Compares inventory list to items being packed. Asks resident to sign if all items are there.		
7.	Puts items to be taken onto the cart, and asks another staff member to help transport items to the pick-up area.		
8.	Helps resident dress in clothing of his choice. Makes sure nurse has removed all dressings, IVs, and tubes that need to be removed prior to discharge.		
9.	Locks wheelchair or stretcher wheels. Helps him safely into the wheelchair or onto stretcher.		
10.	Helps resident say his goodbyes to other residents and the staff.		
11.	Takes him to the pick-up area. Locks wheelchair or stretcher wheels. Helps resident into vehicle. Transfers personal items into the vehicle.		
12.	Says goodbye to resident.		
13.	Washes hands.		
14.	Documents procedure using facility guidelines.		

_____ _____
Date Reviewed   Instructor Signature
_____ _____
Date Performed   Instructor Signature

10
Bedmaking and Unit Care

Making a closed bed

		yes	no
1.	Washes hands.		
2.	If resident is in room, identifies self by name. Identifies resident. Greets resident by name.		
3.	Explains procedure to resident. Speaks clearly, slowly, and directly. Maintains face-to-face contact whenever possible.		
4.	Places clean linen on clean surface within reach (e.g., bedside stand, overbed table, or chair).		
5.	Adjusts bed to a safe level, usually waist high. Locks bed wheels.		
6.	Puts on gloves.		
7.	Loosens and rolls used linen (soiled side inside) from head to foot of bed. Avoids contact with skin or clothes. Places it in a hamper or linen bag. Does not place on overbed table, chair, or floor. Removes pillows and pillowcases and places pillowcases in hamper or bag.		
8.	Removes and discards gloves. Washes hands.		
9.	Remakes bed. Places mattress pad (if using) on the bed.		
10.	Places bottom sheet on bed without shaking linen.		
11.	Makes hospital, or mitered, corners to keep bottom sheet wrinkle-free.		
12.	Puts on disposable absorbent pad and then the draw sheet (if used) in the center of the bed on the bottom sheet. Smoothes, and tightly tucks the bottom sheet and draw sheet together under the sides of bed. Moves from head of the bed to the foot of the bed.		
13.	Places top sheet over bed and centers it.		
14.	Places blanket over bed and centers it.		
15.	Places bedspread over bed and centers it.		
16.	Tucks top sheet and blanket under the foot of the bed and makes hospital corners.		
17.	Folds down the top sheet to make a cuff of about six inches over the blanket.		
18.	Takes a pillow, and with one hand, grasps clean pillowcase at the closed end. Turns it inside out over arm. Using the hand that has the pillowcase over it, grasps one narrow edge of pillow. Pulls pillowcase over it with free hand. Does the same for any other pillows. Places them at head of the bed with open end away from the door.		
19.	Returns bed to lowest position.		
20.	Leaves call light within resident's reach.		
21.	Washes hands.		
22.	Takes laundry bag or hamper to proper area.		
23.	Documents procedure using facility guidelines.		

Date Reviewed _____ Instructor Signature

Date Performed _____ Instructor Signature

Making an open bed

		yes	no
1.	Washes hands.		
2.	Makes a closed bed.		
3.	Stands at head of bed. Grasps top sheet, blanket, and bedspread and folds them down to the foot of the bed. Then brings them back up bed to form a large cuff.		

4.	Brings cuff on the top linens to a point where it is one hand-width above the linen underneath.		
5.	Makes sure all linen is wrinkle-free.		
6.	Washes hands.		
7.	Documents procedure using facility guidelines.		

_____   _____
Date Reviewed   Instructor Signature

_____   _____
Date Performed   Instructor Signature

Making an occupied bed

		yes	no
1.	Identifies self by name. Identifies resident. Greets resident by name.		
2.	Washes hands.		
3.	Explains procedure to resident. Speaks clearly, slowly, and directly. Maintains face-to-face contact whenever possible.		
4.	Provides for resident's privacy with a curtain, screen, or door.		
5.	Places clean linen on clean surface within reach (e.g., bedside stand, overbed table, or chair).		
6.	Adjusts bed to safe working level, usually waist high. Lowers head of bed. Locks bed wheels.		
7.	Puts on gloves.		
8.	Loosens top linen from the end of the bed on the working side.		
9.	Unfolds bath blanket over top sheet and removes the top sheet. Keeps resident covered at all times with the bath blanket.		
10.	Raises bed rail (if bed has them) on far side of bed. Goes to other side of the bed. Helps resident to turn onto her side slowly, moving away from self, toward raised rail.		

11.	Loosens bottom used linen, mattress pad, and absorbent pad on the working side.		
12.	Rolls bottom used linen toward resident and center of bed, soiled side inside. Tucks it snugly against resident's back.		
13.	Places mattress pad (if used) on the bed, attaching elastic at corners on working side.		
14.	Places clean bottom linen or fitted bottom sheet with the center crease in the center. Makes hospital corners to keep bottom sheet wrinkle-free or attaches corners if using fitted sheet.		
15.	Smoothes bottom sheet out toward resident. Makes sure there are no wrinkles in the mattress pad. Rolls extra material toward resident. Tucks it under resident's body.		
16.	If using a disposable absorbent pad, unfolds it and centers it on the bed. Smoothes it out toward resident. Tucks it under resident's body.		
17.	If using a draw sheet, places it on bed. Tucks in on side closest to self and smoothes and tucks.		
18.	Raises bed rail nearest self. Goes to the other side of bed. Lowers bed rail on working side. Helps resident roll or turn onto clean bottom sheet.		
19.	Loosens used linen. Looks for personal items. Rolls linen from head to foot of bed, avoiding contact with skin or clothes. Does not shake used linen. Places it in a hamper or linen bag. Does not place on overbed table, chair, or floor.		

20.	Pulls clean linen through as quickly as possible. Starts with the mattress pad and wraps around corners. Pulls and tucks in clean bottom linen, just like the other side. Pulls and tucks in disposable absorbent pad and draw sheet if used. Makes hospital corners with bottom sheet. Finishes with bottom sheet free of wrinkles.		
21.	Asks resident to turn on his back. Keeps resident covered and comfortable, with a pillow under his head. Raises side rail nearest self.		
22.	Unfolds top sheet. Places it over resident and centers it. Asks resident to hold the top sheet and pulls the bath blanket out from underneath. Puts it in the hamper or bag.		
23.	Places blanket over the top sheet and centers it. Places bedspread over the blanket and centers it. Tucks top sheet, blanket, and bedspread under foot of bed and makes hospital corners on each side. Loosens top linens over resident's feet.		
24.	At the top of the bed, folds down the top sheet to make a cuff of about six inches over blanket.		
25.	Holds and lifts resident's head and removes pillow. Removes used pillowcase by turning it inside out. Places it in hamper or bag.		
26.	Removes and discards gloves. Washes hands.		

27.	Takes a pillow, and with one hand, grasps clean pillowcase at the closed end. Turns it inside out over arm. Using the hand that has the pillowcase over it, grasps one narrow edge of pillow. Pulls pillowcase over it with free hand. Does the same for any other pillows. Places them at head of the bed with open end away from the door.		
28.	Makes sure bed is wrinkle-free. Makes resident comfortable.		
29.	Returns bed to lowest position. Leaves bed rails in ordered position. Removes privacy measures.		
30.	Leaves call light within resident's reach.		
31.	Is courteous and respectful at all times.		
32.	Washes hands.		
33.	Takes laundry bag or hamper to proper area.		
34.	Reports any changes in resident to the nurse. Documents procedure using facility guidelines.		

_____   _____
Date Reviewed   Instructor Signature

_____   _____
Date Performed   Instructor Signature

Making a surgical bed

		yes	no
1.	Washes hands.		
2.	Places clean linen on clean surface within reach (e.g., bedside stand, overbed table, or chair).		
3.	Adjusts bed to safe working level, usually waist high. Locks bed wheels.		
4.	Puts on gloves.		

5.	Removes all used linen, rolling it (soiled side inside) from head to foot of bed. Avoids contact with skin or clothes. Places it in a hamper or linen bag.		
6.	Removes and discards gloves.		
7.	Washes hands.		
8.	Makes a closed bed. Does not tuck top linens under mattress.		
9.	Folds top linens down from the head of the bed and up from the foot of the bed.		
10.	Forms a triangle with the linen. Fanfolds linen triangle into pleated layers and positions opposite the stretcher side of the bed. After fanfolding, forms a tiny tip with the end of linen triangle.		
11.	Puts on clean pillowcases. Places clean pillows on a clean surface off the bed, such as on the bedside stand or chair.		
12.	Leaves bed in its locked position. Leaves both bed rails down.		
13.	Moves all furniture to make room for the stretcher.		
14.	Does not place call light on bed.		
15.	Washes hands.		
16.	Takes laundry bag or hamper to proper area.		
17.	Documents procedure using facility guidelines.		

_____   _____
Date Reviewed   Instructor Signature

_____   _____
Date Performed   Instructor Signature

11
Positioning, Moving, and Lifting

Assisting a resident to move up in bed with assistance (using assist device)		
		yes	no
1.	Identifies self by name. Identifies resident. Greets resident by name.		
2.	Washes hands.		
3.	Explains procedure to resident. Speaks clearly, slowly, and directly. Maintains face-to-face contact whenever possible.		
4.	Provides for resident's privacy with a curtain, screen, or door.		
5.	Adjusts bed to a safe level, usually waist high. Locks bed wheels.		
6.	Lowers head of bed to make it flat. Moves pillow to head of bed.		
7.	Stands on opposite side of bed from helper. Each person is turned slightly toward the head of the bed. Foot that is closest to the head of the bed is pointed in that direction. Stands with feet shoulder-width apart. Bends knees. Keeps back straight.		
8.	Rolls assist device up to resident's side. Has helper do the same on his side of the bed. Grasps sheet with palms up at resident's shoulders and hips. Has helper do the same.		
9.	Shifts weight to back foot. Has helper do the same. On the count of three, shifts weight to forward feet. Slides assist device and resident toward head of bed.		
10.	Places pillow under resident's head.		
11.	Makes resident comfortable. Unrolls draw sheet. Leaves it in place for next repositioning. If using another type of assist device, removes it.		

12.	Returns bed to lowest position. Removes privacy measures.		
13.	Leaves call light within resident's reach.		
14.	Washes hands.		
15.	Is courteous and respectful at all times.		
16.	Reports any changes in resident to the nurse. Documents procedure using facility guidelines.		

_____ _____
Date Reviewed   Instructor Signature

_____ _____
Date Performed   Instructor Signature

13.	Returns bed to lowest position. Removes privacy measures.		
14.	Leaves call light within resident's reach.		
15.	Washes hands.		
16.	Is courteous and respectful at all times.		
17.	Reports any changes in resident to the nurse. Documents procedure using facility guidelines.		

_____ _____
Date Reviewed   Instructor Signature

_____ _____
Date Performed   Instructor Signature

Moving a resident to the side of the bed

		yes	no
1.	Identifies self by name. Identifies resident. Greets resident by name.		
2.	Washes hands.		
3.	Explains procedure to resident. Speaks clearly, slowly, and directly. Maintains face-to-face contact whenever possible.		
4.	Provides for resident's privacy with a curtain, screen, or door.		
5.	Adjusts bed to a safe level, usually waist high. Locks bed wheels.		
6.	Lowers head of bed.		
7.	Stands on same side of bed to which resident is being moved.		
8.	Stands with feet shoulder-width apart. Bends knees. Keeps back straight.		
9.	Slides hands under resident's head and shoulders and moves them toward self.		
10.	Slides hands under resident's midsection and moves it toward self.		
11.	Slides hands under resident's hips and legs and moves them toward self.		
12.	Makes resident comfortable.		

Moving a resident to the side of the bed with assistance (using assist device)

		yes	no
1.	Identifies self by name. Identifies resident. Greets resident by name.		
2.	Washes hands.		
3.	Explains procedure to resident. Speaks clearly, slowly, and directly. Maintains face-to-face contact whenever possible.		
4.	Provides for resident's privacy with a curtain, screen, or door.		
5.	Adjusts bed to a safe level, usually waist high. Locks bed wheels.		
6.	Lowers head of bed. Moves pillow to head of bed.		
7.	Stands on opposite side of bed from helper, facing helper. Stands up straight, facing side of bed, with feet shoulder-width apart. Points feet toward side of bed. Bends knees.		
8.	Rolls assist device up to resident's side. Has helper do the same on his side of the bed. Grasps sheet with palms up at resident's shoulders and hips. Has helper do the same.		
9.	On the count of three, slides resident toward side of bed, with weight equal on each foot.		

10.	Places pillow under resident's head.		
11.	Makes resident comfortable. Unrolls draw sheet. Leaves it in place for the next repositioning. If using another type of assist device, removes it.		
12.	Returns bed to lowest position. Removes privacy measures.		
13.	Leaves call light within resident's reach.		
14.	Washes hands.		
15.	Is courteous and respectful at all times.		
16.	Reports any changes in resident to the nurse. Documents procedure using facility guidelines.		

_____   _____
Date Reviewed   Instructor Signature

_____   _____
Date Performed   Instructor Signature

Turning a resident toward you

		yes	no
1.	Identifies self by name. Identifies resident. Greets resident by name.		
2.	Washes hands.		
3.	Explains procedure to resident. Speaks clearly, slowly, and directly. Maintains face-to-face contact whenever possible.		
4.	Provides for resident's privacy with a curtain, screen, or door.		
5.	Adjusts bed to a safe level, usually waist high. Locks bed wheels.		
6.	Lowers head of bed.		
7.	Raises far bed rail.		
8.	Moves resident to far side of bed.		
9.	Crosses resident's arm over his chest. Moves arm on side resident is being turned to out of the way. Crosses far leg over the near leg.		

10.	Stands with feet shoulder-width apart. Bends knees.		
11.	Places one hand on resident's far shoulder. Places other hand on the resident's far hip.		
12.	Supports resident's body. Rolls resident toward self as a unit. Makes sure resident's face is not covered by pillow.		
13.	Positions resident properly:		
	• Head supported by pillow (resident's face should not be obstructed by pillow)		
	• Shoulder adjusted so resident is not lying on arm		
	• Top arm supported by pillow		
	• Back supported by supportive device		
	• Hips properly aligned		
	• Supportive device between legs with top knee flexed; knee and ankle supported		
	• Pillow under bottom foot so that toes are not touching the bed		
14.	Covers resident with top linens. Makes resident comfortable.		
15.	Returns bed to lowest position. Returns bed rails to ordered position. Removes privacy measures.		
16.	Leaves call light within resident's reach.		
17.	Washes hands.		
18.	Is courteous and respectful at all times.		
19.	Reports any changes in resident to the nurse. Documents procedure using facility guidelines.		

_____   _____
Date Reviewed   Instructor Signature

_____   _____
Date Performed   Instructor Signature

Name: _____

Logrolling a resident with assistance

		yes	no
1.	Identifies self by name. Identifies resident. Greets resident by name.		
2.	Washes hands.		
3.	Explains procedure to resident. Speaks clearly, slowly, and directly. Maintains face-to-face contact whenever possible.		
4.	Provides for resident's privacy with a curtain, screen, or door.		
5.	Adjusts bed to a safe level, usually waist high. Locks bed wheels.		
6.	Lowers head of bed.		
7.	With both workers on same side of bed, stands at resident's head and shoulders. Helper stands near resident's midsection.		
8.	Places pillow under resident's head to support neck during move.		
9.	Places resident's arms across his chest. Places pillow between the knees.		
10.	Stands with feet shoulder-width apart. Bends knees.		
11.	Grasps assist device on the far side.		
12.	On the count of three, rolls resident toward self, turning as a unit.		
13.	Repositions resident comfortably in proper alignment. Unrolls draw sheet. Leaves it in place for the next repositioning or removes if using another type of device. Covers resident with top linens.		
14.	Returns bed to lowest position. Removes privacy measures.		
15.	Leaves call light within resident's reach.		
16.	Washes hands.		

		yes	no
17.	Is courteous and respectful at all times.		
18.	Reports any changes in resident to the nurse. Documents procedure using facility guidelines.		

_____   _____
Date Reviewed   Instructor Signature

_____   _____
Date Performed   Instructor Signature

Assisting a resident to sit up on the side of the bed: dangling

		yes	no
1.	Identifies self by name. Identifies resident. Greets resident by name.		
2.	Washes hands.		
3.	Explains procedure to resident. Speaks clearly, slowly, and directly. Maintains face-to-face contact whenever possible.		
4.	Provides for resident's privacy with a curtain, screen, or door.		
5.	Adjusts bed to lowest position. Locks bed wheels.		
6.	Raises head of bed to sitting position. Folds linen to the foot of the bed.		
7.	Stands at side of bed with feet shoulder-width apart. Bends knees. Keeps back straight. Helps resident slowly move toward self.		
8.	Places one arm under resident's shoulder blades. Places other arm under resident's thighs.		
9.	On the count of three, turns resident into sitting position with legs dangling over the side of bed.		
10.	Asks resident to sit up straight and hold onto edge of mattress. Assists resident to put on non-skid shoes if he is going to get out of bed.		
11.	Has resident dangle as long as ordered.		

12.	Takes vital signs as ordered.		
13.	Removes shoes.		
14.	Assists resident back into bed. Places one arm around resident's shoulders. Places other arm under resident's knees. Moves resident's legs onto bed.		
15.	Makes resident comfortable. Covers resident with top linens. Replaces pillow under resident's head.		
16.	Leaves bed in lowest position. Removes privacy measures.		
17.	Leaves call light within resident's reach.		
18.	Washes hands.		
19.	Is courteous and respectful at all times.		
20.	Reports any changes in resident to the nurse. Documents procedure using facility guidelines.		

Date Reviewed _____ Instructor Signature _____

Date Performed _____ Instructor Signature _____

Applying a transfer belt

		yes	no
1.	Identifies self by name. Identifies resident. Greets resident by name.		
2.	Washes hands.		
3.	Explains procedure to resident. Speaks clearly, slowly, and directly. Maintains face-to-face contact whenever possible.		
4.	Provides for resident's privacy with a curtain, screen, or door.		
5.	Adjusts bed to lowest position. Locks bed wheels.		
6.	Supporting the back and hips, assists resident to a sitting position with feet flat on the floor.		
7.	Puts nonskid footwear on resident and fastens.		

8.	Places belt over resident's clothing below the rib cage and above the waist. Does not put it over bare skin.		
9.	Tightens buckle until it is snug. Leaves enough room to insert flat fingers under the belt.		
10.	Checks to make sure that skin or skin folds are not caught under belt.		
11.	Positions buckle slightly off-center in the front or back for comfort.		

Date Reviewed _____ Instructor Signature _____

Date Performed _____ Instructor Signature _____

Transferring a resident from a bed to a chair or wheelchair

		yes	no
1.	Identifies self by name. Identifies resident. Greets resident by name.		
2.	Washes hands.		
3.	Explains procedure to resident. Speaks clearly, slowly, and directly. Maintains face-to-face contact whenever possible.		
4.	Provides for resident's privacy with a curtain, screen, or door.		
5.	Places wheelchair at the head of the bed, facing the foot of the bed, or at the foot of bed, facing the head of bed. Places wheelchair on resident's stronger side.		
6.	Removes wheelchair footrests close to the bed.		
7.	Locks wheelchair wheels.		
8.	Raises head of bed. Adjusts bed level to lowest position. Locks bed wheels.		
9.	Assists resident to a sitting position with feet flat on the floor.		
10.	Puts nonskid footwear on resident and fastens.		

164

Name: _____

11.	Stands in front of resident. Stands with feet about shoulder-width apart. Bends knees. Keeps back straight.		
12.	Places transfer belt around resident's waist over clothing (not on bare skin). Tightens buckle until it is snug. Grasps belt securely on both sides, with hands in an upward position.		
13.	Provides instructions to allow resident to help with transfer.		
14.	With legs, braces resident's lower legs to prevent slipping.		
15.	On the count of three, with hands still grasping the transfer belt on both sides and moving upward, helps resident to stand.		
16.	Tells resident to take small steps in the direction of the chair while turning her back toward the chair. Helps pivot resident toward chair if more help is needed.		
17.	Asks resident to put hands on wheelchair armrests if able. When the resident's legs touch the back of the chair, helps her lower herself into chair.		
18.	Repositions resident with hips touching back of wheelchair.		
19.	Attaches footrests. Places resident's feet on footrests. Checks that resident is in proper alignment. Removes transfer belt.		
20.	Makes resident comfortable.		
21.	Leaves bed in lowest position. Removes privacy measures.		
22.	Leaves call light within resident's reach.		
23.	Washes hands.		
24.	Is courteous and respectful at all times.		
25.	Reports any changes in resident to the nurse. Documents procedure using facility guidelines.		

	To transfer back to bed from a wheelchair:		
1.	Performs steps 1 through 7 above.		
2.	Adjusts bed level to a low position, with height of bed equal to or slightly lower than the chair. Locks bed wheels.		
3.	Performs steps 11 through 15 above.		
4.	Helps resident pivot to bed with back of resident's legs against bed. When resident feels the bed, he slowly sits down on the side of the bed.		
5.	Removes transfer belt. Removes footwear. Makes resident comfortable.		
6.	Returns bed to lowest position. Removes privacy measures.		
7.	Leaves call light within resident's reach.		
8.	Washes hands.		
9.	Is courteous and respectful at all times.		
10.	Reports any changes in resident to the nurse. Documents procedure using facility guidelines.		

_____ _____
Date Reviewed   Instructor Signature

_____ _____
Date Performed   Instructor Signature

Transferring a resident from a bed to a stretcher with assistance

		yes	no
1.	Identifies self by name. Identifies resident. Greets resident by name.		
2.	Washes hands.		
3.	Explains procedure to resident. Speaks clearly, slowly, and directly. Maintains face-to-face contact whenever possible.		
4.	Provides for resident's privacy with a curtain, screen, or door.		

5.	Lowers head of bed so that it is flat. Locks bed wheels.		
6.	Folds linens to foot of the bed. Covers resident with bath blanket.		
7.	Moves resident to the side of bed.		
8.	Places stretcher solidly against bed, with bed height equal to or slightly above height of stretcher. Locks stretcher wheels. Moves stretcher safety belts out of the way.		
9.	Two workers are on the side of the bed opposite the stretcher. Two more workers are on the other side of the stretcher.		
10.	Each worker rolls up the sides of the draw sheet and prepares to move resident.		
11.	On the count of three, all workers lift and move resident to stretcher.		
12.	Raises head of stretcher or places a pillow under resident's head. Makes sure resident is still covered.		
13.	Secures safety belts across resident. Raises bed rails on stretcher.		
14.	Unlocks stretcher's wheels. Takes resident to proper site. Stays with the resident until another team member takes over responsibility of the resident.		
15.	Washes hands.		
16.	Is courteous and respectful at all times.		
17.	Reports any changes in resident to the nurse. Documents procedure using facility guidelines.		

_____   _____
Date Reviewed   Instructor Signature

_____   _____
Date Performed   Instructor Signature

Transferring a resident using a mechanical lift with assistance

		yes	no
1.	Identifies self by name. Identifies resident. Greets resident by name.		
2.	Washes hands.		
3.	Explains procedure to resident. Speaks clearly, slowly, and directly. Maintains face-to-face contact whenever possible.		
4.	Provides for resident's privacy with a curtain, screen, or door.		
5.	Adjusts bed to a safe level, usually waist high. Locks bed wheels.		
6.	Positions wheelchair next to bed. Removes wheelchair footrests close to the bed. Locks wheelchair wheels.		
7.	Helps resident turn toward self. Pads the sling where the neck will rest with a washcloth for resident's comfort. Fanfolds sling if possible. Makes bottom of sling even with the resident's knees. Helps resident roll onto his back. Spreads out fanfolded edge of the sling.		
8.	Rolls mechanical lift to bedside. Makes sure the base is opened to its widest point. Pushes base of the lift under bed. Locks lift wheels.		
9.	Places overhead bar directly over resident.		
10.	With the resident lying on his back, attaches one set of straps to each side of the sling. Attaches one set of straps to overhead bar. Has coworker support the resident at the head, shoulders, and knees while being lifted. Makes sure all straps are connected properly.		

Name: _____

		yes	no
11.	Following manufacturer's instructions, raises resident two inches above the bed. Pauses a moment for the resident to regain balance. Unlocks lift wheels.		
12.	Has coworker support and guide resident's body until resident is positioned over the chair or wheelchair.		
13.	Lowers resident into chair or wheelchair. Pushes down gently on resident's knees to help resident into a sitting position.		
14.	Undoes straps from overhead bar. Leaves sling in place or removes it.		
15.	Makes sure resident is seated comfortably and correctly in the chair or wheelchair. Puts nonskid footwear on resident and fastens. Attaches footrests and places resident's feet on footrests.		
16.	Returns bed to lowest position. Removes privacy measures.		
17.	Leaves call light within resident's reach.		
18.	Washes hands.		
19.	Is courteous and respectful at all times.		
20.	Reports any changes in resident to the nurse. Documents procedure using facility guidelines.		

_____ _____
Date Reviewed   Instructor Signature

_____ _____
Date Performed   Instructor Signature

Transferring a resident onto and off of a toilet

		yes	no
1.	Identifies self by name. Identifies resident. Greets resident by name.		
2.	Washes hands.		
3.	Explains procedure to resident. Speaks clearly, slowly, and directly. Maintains face-to-face contact whenever possible.		
4.	Provides for resident's privacy with a curtain, screen, or door.		
5.	Positions wheelchair at a right angle to the toilet to face hand bar/wall rail. Places wheelchair on resident's stronger side.		
6.	Removes wheelchair footrests. Locks wheels.		
7.	Puts on gloves.		
8.	Applies a transfer belt around the resident's waist over clothing (not on bare skin). Grasps the belt securely on both sides, with hands in an upward position.		
9.	Asks resident to push against the armrests of the wheelchair and stand, reaching for and grasping the hand bar with her stronger arm. Moves wheelchair out of the way.		
10.	Asks resident to pivot her feet and back up so that she can feel the front of the toilet with the back of her legs.		
11.	Helps resident to pull down pants and underwear.		
12.	Helps resident to slowly sit down onto the toilet. Gives privacy unless resident cannot be left alone. Removes and discards gloves. Washes hands. Closes bathroom door. Stays near the door until resident is finished.		
13.	When called, returns and dons clean gloves. Assists with perineal care as necessary. Asks her to stand and reach for the hand bar.		
14.	Uses toilet paper or wipes to clean the resident. Makes sure she is clean and dry before pulling up clothing. Removes and discards gloves.		

15.	Helps resident to the sink to wash hands.		
16.	Washes hands.		
17.	Helps resident back into wheelchair. Makes sure the resident is seated comfortably and correctly in the wheelchair. Removes transfer belt. Replaces footrests.		
18.	Helps resident to leave the bathroom.		
19.	Leaves call light within resident's reach.		
20.	Washes hands.		
21.	Is courteous and respectful at all times.		
22.	Reports any changes in resident to the nurse. Documents procedure using facility guidelines.		

_____   _____
Date Reviewed   Instructor Signature

_____   _____
Date Performed   Instructor Signature

Transferring a resident into a vehicle

		yes	no
1.	Identifies self by name. Identifies resident. Greets resident by name.		
2.	Washes hands.		
3.	Explains procedure to resident. Speaks clearly, slowly, and directly. Maintains face-to-face contact whenever possible.		
4.	Places wheelchair close to the vehicle at a 45-degree angle. Opens door on the resident's stronger side if possible.		
5.	Locks wheelchair wheels.		
6.	Asks resident to push against armrests of the wheelchair and stand. Asks resident to stand, grasp the vehicle or dashboard, and pivot his foot so the side of the seat touches the back of the legs.		

7.	Has resident sit in the seat and lift one leg, and then the other, into the vehicle.		
8.	Positions resident comfortably in the vehicle. Helps fasten seat belt.		
9.	Has coworker place belongings in vehicle. Shuts the door(s).		
10.	Returns wheelchair and cart to appropriate place for cleaning.		
11.	Washes hands.		
12.	Documents procedure using facility guidelines.		

_____   _____
Date Reviewed   Instructor Signature

_____   _____
Date Performed   Instructor Signature

Assisting a resident to ambulate

		yes	no
1.	Identifies self by name. Identifies resident. Greets resident by name.		
2.	Washes hands.		
3.	Explains procedure to resident. Speaks clearly, slowly, and directly. Maintains face-to-face contact whenever possible.		
4.	Provides for resident's privacy with a curtain, screen, or door.		
5.	Adjusts bed to lowest position. Locks bed wheels. Assists resident to sitting position with his feet flat on the floor.		
6.	Puts nonskid footwear on resident and fastens.		
7.	Stands in front of and faces resident. Stands with feet shoulder-width apart. Bends knees. Keeps back straight.		

8.	Places transfer belt around the resident's waist over clothing (not on bare skin). Checks to make sure that skin or skin folds (for example, breasts) are not caught under the belt. Grasps the belt securely on both sides, with hands in an upward position.		
9.	If resident is unable to stand without help, braces (supports) the resident's lower extremities.		
10.	On the count of three, with hands still grasping the transfer belt on both sides and moving upward, helps resident to stand.		
11.	Walks slightly behind and to one side of resident for the full distance, while holding onto the transfer belt. If the resident has a weaker side, stands on the weaker side. Asks resident to look forward, not down at floor, during ambulation.		
12.	After ambulation, removes transfer belt. Makes resident comfortable. Removes footwear.		
13.	Leaves bed in lowest position. Removes privacy measures.		
14.	Leaves call light within resident's reach.		
15.	Washes hands.		
16.	Is courteous and respectful at all times.		
17.	Reports any changes in resident to the nurse. Documents procedure using facility guidelines.		

_____   _____
Date Reviewed   Instructor Signature

_____   _____
Date Performed   Instructor Signature

12
Personal Care

Giving a complete bed bath			
		yes	no
1.	Identifies self by name. Identifies resident. Greets resident by name.		
2.	Washes hands.		
3.	Explains procedure to resident. Speaks clearly, slowly, and directly. Maintains face-to-face contact whenever possible.		
4.	Provides for resident's privacy with a curtain, screen, or door.		
5.	Adjusts bed to a safe level, usually waist high. Locks bed wheels.		
6.	Places a bath blanket or towel over resident. Asks him to hold onto it as bedding is folded back. Removes gown, while keeping resident covered with bath blanket or top sheet.		
7.	Fills basin with warm water. Tests water temperature with thermometer or wrist and ensures it is safe. Has resident check water temperature. Adjusts if necessary. Changes water when it becomes too cool, soapy, or dirty.		
8.	Puts on gloves.		
9.	Asks resident to participate in washing.		
10.	Uncovers only one part of body at a time. Places towel under the body part being washed.		
11.	Washes, rinses, and dries one part of the body at a time. Starts at head. Works down, and completes the front first. When washing, uses a clean area of the washcloth for each stroke.		

Eyes, Face, Ears, Neck: Washes face with wet washcloth (no soap). Begins with the eye farther away from self. Washes inner area to outer area. Uses a different area of the washcloth for each eye. Washes face from the middle outward. Washes ears and behind the ears and the neck. Rinses and pats dry with blotting motion.		
Arms and Axillae: Removes far arm from under the towel. With a soapy washcloth, washes upper arm and underarm. Uses long strokes from the shoulder to the wrist. Rinses and pats dry. Repeats for the other arm.		
Hands: Washes far hand in a basin. Cleans under the nails with an orangewood stick or nail brush. Rinses and pats dry. Makes sure to dry between the fingers. Gives nail care. Repeats for the other hand. Puts lotion on the resident's elbows and hands if ordered.		
Chest: Places towel across resident's chest. Pulls bath blanket down to the waist. Lifts the towel only enough to wash the chest. Rinses it and pats dry. For a female resident, washes, rinses, and dries breasts and under breasts. Checks skin in this area for signs of irritation.		
Abdomen: Keeps towel across chest. Folds bath blanket down so that it still covers the genital area. Washes abdomen, rinses, and pats dry. Covers with towel. Pulls bath blanket up to the resident's chin. Removes towel.		
Legs and Feet: Exposes far leg. Places towel under it. Washes thigh, using downward strokes. Rinses and pats dry. Does the same from knee to ankle.		

	Places another towel under the far foot. Moves basin to the towel. Places foot into basin. Washes foot and between the toes. Rinses foot and pats dry. Dries between toes. Gives nail care if it has been assigned. Applies lotion to the foot if ordered, especially at the heels. Does not apply lotion between the toes. Removes excess lotion. Repeats steps for the other leg and foot.		
	Back: Helps resident move to center of the bed. Asks resident to turn onto his side so his back is facing self. If the bed has rails, raises rail on the far side for safety. Folds blanket away from the back. Places a towel lengthwise next to the back. Washes the back, neck, and buttocks with long, downward strokes. Rinses and pats dry. Applies lotion if ordered.		
12.	Places towel under the buttocks and upper thighs. Helps the resident turn onto his back. If the resident is able to wash his or her perineal area, places a basin of clean, warm water and a washcloth and towel within reach. Hands items to the resident as needed. Removes and discards gloves, washes hands, leaves bed rails up, and lowers bed if asked to leave the room. Leaves supplies and the call light within reach. If the resident has a urinary catheter in place, reminds him not to pull on it.		
13.	If the resident cannot do perineal care by himself, removes and discards gloves. Washes hands. Puts on clean gloves.		
14.	Covers resident with bath blanket. Removes pad or towel and places it in proper container.		

Name: _____

15.	Empties, rinses, and dries bath basin. Places basin in designated dirty supply area or returns to storage, depending on policy.		
16.	Places used clothing and linens in proper containers.		
17.	Removes and discards gloves.		
18.	Washes hands.		
19.	Provides deodorant. Puts clean gown or clothes on resident. Assists with brushing or combing resident's hair.		
20.	Replaces bedding. Places the bath blanket in the proper container. Makes resident comfortable.		
21.	Returns bed to lowest position. Removes privacy measures.		
22.	Leaves call light within resident's reach.		
23.	Washes hands.		
24.	Is courteous and respectful at all times.		
25.	Reports any changes in resident to the nurse. Documents procedure using facility guidelines.		

_____   _____
Date Reviewed   Instructor Signature

_____   _____
Date Performed   Instructor Signature

Providing perineal care

		yes	no
1.	Identifies self by name. Identifies resident. Greets resident by name.		
2.	Washes hands.		
3.	Explains procedure to resident. Speaks clearly, slowly, and directly. Maintains face-to-face contact whenever possible.		
4.	Provides for resident's privacy with a curtain, screen, or door.		
5.	Adjusts bed to a safe level, usually waist high. Locks bed wheels.		
6.	Places a bath blanket or towel over resident. Asks him to hold onto it as bedding is folded back. Removes undergarments, while keeping resident covered with bath blanket or top sheet. Places clothing in hamper.		
7.	Fills basin with warm water. Tests water temperature with thermometer or wrist and ensures it is safe. Has resident check water temperature. Adjusts if necessary. Changes water when it becomes too cool, soapy, or dirty.		
8.	Puts on gloves.		
9.	Places a towel or absorbent pad under the perineal area.		
10.	Works from front to back (clean to dirty).		
	For a female resident: Uses water and a small amount of soap, and cleans from front to back. Uses single strokes. Uses a clean area of washcloth or clean washcloth for each stroke.		
	Separates the labia majora and wipes from front to back on one side with a clean washcloth, using a single stroke. Using a clean area of the washcloth, wipes the other side from front to back. Using another clean area of the washcloth, wipes down the center from front to back. Cleans the perineum (area between genitals and anus) last with a front to back motion. Rinses the area thoroughly in the same way. Makes sure all soap is removed.		

	Dries entire perineal area. Moves from front to back. Asks resident to turn on her side. Washes, rinses, and dries buttocks and anal area. Cleans anal area without contaminating the perineal area.		
	For a male resident: If the resident is uncircumcised, pulls back the foreskin first. Pushes skin toward the base of penis. Holds penis by the shaft. Washes in a circular motion from the tip down to the base. Uses clean area of washcloth or clean washcloth for each stroke.		
	Thoroughly rinses the penis. If resident is uncircumcised, returns foreskin to normal position. Then washes scrotum and groin. Rinses thoroughly and pats dry. Asks resident to turn on his side. Washes, rinses, and dries buttocks and anal area. Cleans anal area without contaminating the perineal area.		
11.	Covers the resident with the bath blanket. Removes absorbent pad or towel and places in proper container.		
12.	Empties, rinses, and dries bath basin. Places basin in designated dirty supply area or returns to storage, depending on policy.		
13.	Places used clothing and linens in proper containers.		
14.	Removes and discards gloves. Washes hands.		
15.	Helps resident put on clean undergarment. Replaces bedding. Places the bath blanket in the proper container. Makes resident comfortable.		
16.	Returns bed to lowest position. Removes privacy measures.		
17.	Leaves call light within resident's reach.		

18.	Washes hands.		
19.	Is courteous and respectful at all times.		
20.	Reports any changes in resident to the nurse. Documents procedure using facility guidelines.		

_____ _____
Date Reviewed   Instructor Signature

_____ _____
Date Performed   Instructor Signature

Shampooing a resident's hair in bed

		yes	no
1.	Identifies self by name. Identifies resident. Greets resident by name.		
2.	Washes hands.		
3.	Explains procedure to resident. Speaks clearly, slowly, and directly. Maintains face-to-face contact whenever possible.		
4.	Provides for resident's privacy with a curtain, screen, or door.		
5.	Arranges supplies within reach.		
6.	Tests water temperature with thermometer or wrist and ensures it is safe. Has resident check water temperature. Adjusts if necessary.		
7.	Removes pillows and places resident in flat position. Adjusts bed to a safe level, usually waist high. Locks bed wheels.		
8.	Puts on gloves.		
9.	Places waterproof pad under resident's head and shoulders. Covers resident with the bath blanket. Folds back the top sheet and regular blankets.		
10.	Places basin under resident's head. Places one towel across the resident's shoulders.		
11.	Protects resident's eyes with dry washcloth.		

12.	Uses pitcher or attachment to wet hair thoroughly. Applies a small amount of shampoo to hands, usually the size of a quarter.		
13.	Lathers and massages scalp with fingertips. Uses a circular motion from front to back.		
14.	Rinses hair until water runs clear. Applies conditioner if requested. Rinses hair thoroughly to prevent the scalp from getting dry and itchy.		
15.	Wraps resident's hair in a clean towel. Removes basin and waterproof pad. Dries face with washcloth used to protect eyes.		
16.	Raises head of bed.		
17.	Rubs scalp and hair with towel. Combs or brushes resident's hair. Dries hair with hair dryer on low. Styles hair as the resident prefers.		
18.	Empties, rinses, and wipes basin/pitcher. Returns to proper storage.		
19.	Cleans comb or brush. Returns hair dryer and comb/brush to proper storage. Places used linen in proper container.		
20.	Removes and discards gloves. Washes hands.		
21.	Makes resident comfortable.		
22.	Returns bed to lowest position. Removes privacy measures.		
23.	Leaves call light within resident's reach.		
24.	Washes hands.		
25.	Is courteous and respectful at all times.		
26.	Reports any changes in resident to the nurse. Documents procedure using facility guidelines.		

_____ _____
Date Reviewed   Instructor Signature

_____ _____
Date Performed   Instructor Signature

Giving a shower or tub bath

		yes	no
1.	Washes hands.		
2.	Places equipment in shower or tub room. Puts on gloves. Cleans shower or tub area and shower chair. Places bucket under shower chair. Turns on heat lamp.		
3.	Removes and discards gloves. Washes hands.		
4.	Goes to resident's room. Identifies self by name. Identifies the resident. Greets the resident by name.		
5.	Explains procedure to resident. Speaks clearly, slowly, and directly. Maintains face-to-face contact whenever possible.		
6.	Provides for resident's privacy with a curtain, screen, or door.		
7.	Helps resident to put on non-skid footwear. Transports resident to shower or tub room, while keeping resident covered.		
8.	Washes hands. Puts on clean gloves.		
9.	Helps resident remove clothing and shoes. Covers residents with bath blanket.		
	For a shower:		
10.	If using a shower chair, places it into position and locks its wheels. Transfers resident into shower chair.		
11.	Turns on water. Tests water temperature with thermometer or wrist. Has resident check water temperature. Adjusts if necessary. Checks water temperature frequently throughout the shower.		
12.	Unlocks shower chair and moves it into the stall. Locks wheels.		

13.	Stays with resident during the entire procedure.		
14.	Lets resident wash as much as possible on his own. Helps to wash as needed.		
15.	Helps resident shampoo hair. Rinses hair thoroughly.		
16.	Helps to wash and rinse the entire body. Moves from head to toe (clean to dirty).		
17.	Turns off water. Unlocks shower chair wheels. Rolls resident out of shower.		
	For a tub bath:		
10.	Transfers resident onto chair or tub lift.		
11.	Fills the tub halfway with warm water. Tests water temperature with thermometer or wrist and ensures it is safe. Has resident check water temperature. Adjusts if necessary.		
12.	Stays with resident during the entire procedure.		
13.	Lets resident wash as much as possible on his own. Helps to wash as needed.		
14.	Helps resident shampoo hair. Rinses hair thoroughly.		
15.	Helps to wash and rinse the entire body. Moves from head to toe (clean to dirty).		
16.	Drains tub. Covers resident with bath blanket while the tub drains.		
17.	Helps resident out of tub and onto a chair.		
	Remaining steps for either procedure:		
18.	Gives resident towel(s) and helps to pat dry everywhere, including under the breasts, between skin folds, in the perineal area, and between toes. Applies lotion and deodorant as needed.		

19.	Places used clothing and linens in proper containers.		
20.	Removes and discards gloves.		
21.	Washes hands.		
22.	Helps resident dress and dry and comb hair before leaving shower or tub room. Puts on nonskid footwear. Returns resident to room.		
23.	Makes resident comfortable.		
24.	Leaves call light within resident's reach.		
25.	Washes hands.		
26.	Is courteous and respectful at all times.		
27.	Reports any changes in resident to the nurse. Documents procedure using facility guidelines.		

Date Reviewed _____   Instructor Signature _____

Date Performed _____   Instructor Signature _____

Giving a back rub

		yes	no
1.	Identifies self by name. Identifies resident. Greets resident by name.		
2.	Washes hands.		
3.	Explains procedure to resident. Speaks clearly, slowly, and directly. Maintains face-to-face contact whenever possible.		
4.	Provides for resident's privacy with a curtain, screen, or door.		
5.	Adjusts bed to a safe level, usually waist high. Lowers head of bed. Locks bed wheels.		
6.	Positions resident lying on his side (lateral position) or his stomach (prone position). Covers with a bath blanket. Exposes back to the top of the buttocks.		

Name: _____

7.	Warms lotion by putting bottle in warm water for five minutes. Runs hands under warm water. Pours lotion on hands. Rubs them together.		
8.	Places hands on each side of upper part of the buttocks. Uses full palm of hand. Makes long, smooth, upward strokes with both hands. Moves along each side of the spine, up to the shoulders. Circles hands outward. Moves back along outer edges of the back. At buttocks, makes another circle. Moves hands back up to the shoulders. Without taking hands from resident's skin, repeats this motion for three to five minutes.		
9.	Kneads with the first two fingers and thumb of each hand. Places them at base of the spine. Moves upward together along each side of the spine. Applies gentle downward pressure with fingers and thumbs. Follows same direction as with the long smooth strokes, circling at shoulders and buttocks.		
10.	Massages bony areas (spine, shoulder blades, hip bones). Uses circular motions of fingertips. Does not massage any pale, white, purple, or red areas.		
11.	Finishes with long, smooth strokes.		
12.	Dries the back if it has extra lotion remaining.		
13.	Removes bath blanket. Helps resident to get dressed. Makes resident comfortable.		
14.	Returns bed to lowest position. Removes privacy measures.		
15.	Stores supplies. Places used clothing and linens in proper containers.		

16.	Leaves call light within resident's reach.		
17.	Washes hands.		
18.	Is courteous and respectful at all times.		
19.	Reports any changes in the resident to the nurse, including pale, white, or red areas. Documents procedure using facility guidelines.		

Date Reviewed _____   Instructor Signature _____

Date Performed _____   Instructor Signature _____

Providing mouth care

		yes	no
1.	Identifies self by name. Identifies resident. Greets resident by name.		
2.	Washes hands.		
3.	Explains procedure to resident. Speaks clearly, slowly, and directly. Maintains face-to-face contact whenever possible.		
4.	Provides for resident's privacy with a curtain, screen, or door.		
5.	Adjusts bed to safe working level, usually waist high. Raises head of bed to make sure resident is sitting upright. Locks bed wheels.		
6.	Puts on gloves.		
7.	Places clothing protector or towel across resident's chest.		
8.	Wets brush. Applies toothpaste.		
9.	Cleans entire mouth, including tongue and all surfaces of teeth and the gumline, using gentle strokes. First brushes inner, outer, and chewing surfaces of the upper teeth, then does the same with the lower teeth. Uses short strokes. Brushes back and forth. Brushes tongue.		

10.	Gives resident water to rinse the mouth. Places emesis basin under the resident's chin, with the inward curve under the chin. Has resident spit water into emesis basin. Wipes resident's mouth and removes protector or towel. Applies lip moisturizer.		
11.	Rinses toothbrush and places in proper container. Empties, rinses, and dries emesis basin. Places basin in designated dirty supply area or returns to storage, depending on facility policy.		
12.	Places used linen in proper container.		
13.	Removes and discards gloves. Washes hands.		
14.	Makes resident comfortable.		
15.	Returns bed to lowest position. Removes privacy measures.		
16.	Leaves call light within resident's reach.		
17.	Washes hands.		
18.	Is courteous and respectful at all times.		
19.	Reports any changes in resident to the nurse. Reports any problems with teeth, mouth, tongue, or lips to nurse. These include odor, cracking, sores, bleeding, and any discoloration. Documents procedure using facility guidelines.		

_____   _____
Date Reviewed   Instructor Signature

_____   _____
Date Performed   Instructor Signature

Flossing teeth

		yes	no
1.	Identifies self by name. Identifies resident. Greets resident by name.		
2.	Washes hands.		
3.	Explains procedure to resident. Speaks clearly, slowly, and directly. Maintains face-to-face contact whenever possible.		
4.	Provides for resident's privacy with a curtain, screen, or door.		
5.	Adjusts bed to safe working level, usually waist high. Raises head of bed to have resident in upright sitting position. Locks bed wheels.		
6.	Puts on gloves.		
7.	Wraps ends of floss securely around each index finger.		
8.	Starting with the back teeth, places floss between teeth. Moves it down the surface of the tooth. Uses a gentle sawing motion.		
	Continues to the gum line. At the gum line, curves the floss. Slips it gently into the space between the gum and tooth. Then goes back up, scraping that side of the tooth. Repeats on the side of the other tooth.		
9.	After every two teeth, unwinds floss from fingers. Moves floss to use a clean area. Flosses all teeth.		
10.	Offers water to rinse the mouth. Asks resident to spit it into the basin.		
11.	Offers resident a face towel when done.		
12.	Discards floss. Discards water in the toilet. Rinses basin and places basin in designated dirty supply area or returns to storage, depending on facility policy. Stores supplies.		
13.	Places used linen in the proper container.		
14.	Removes and discards gloves. Washes hands.		
15.	Makes resident comfortable.		

16.	Returns bed to lowest position. Removes privacy measures.		
17.	Leaves call light within resident's reach.		
18.	Washes hands.		
19.	Is courteous and respectful at all times.		
20.	Reports any changes in resident to the nurse. Reports any problems with teeth, mouth, tongue, or lips to nurse. These include odor, cracking, sores, bleeding, and any discoloration. Documents procedure using facility guidelines.		

_____ _____
Date Reviewed   Instructor Signature

_____ _____
Date Performed   Instructor Signature

Cleaning and storing dentures

		yes	no
1.	Identifies self by name. Identifies resident. Greets resident by name.		
2.	Washes hands.		
3.	Explains procedure to resident. Speaks clearly, slowly, and directly. Maintains face-to-face contact whenever possible.		
4.	Provides for resident's privacy with a curtain, screen, or door.		
5.	Adjusts bed to safe working level, usually waist high. Raises head of bed to make sure resident is sitting upright. Locks bed wheels.		
6.	Puts on gloves.		
7.	Lines sink/basin with towel(s) and partially fills sink with water.		
8.	If removing dentures, removes lower denture first. Grasps lower denture with a gauze square and removes it. Firmly grasps upper denture with a gauze square. Gives a slight downward pull to break the suction. Turns it at an angle to take it out of the mouth.		

9.	Rinses dentures in moderate/cool running water before brushing them.		
10.	Applies cleanser to toothbrush.		
11.	Brushes dentures on all surfaces.		
12.	Rinses all surfaces of dentures under moderate/cool running water.		
13.	Offers water to rinse the resident's mouth. Asks resident to spit it into the emesis basin.		
14.	Rinses denture cup if placing clean dentures inside it.		
15.	Places dentures in clean denture cup with special solution or moderate/cool water and cover. Makes sure cup is labeled with resident's name. Returns denture cup to storage.		
16.	If replacing dentures in resident's mouth, makes sure resident is still sitting upright. Applies denture cream or adhesive to the dentures if needed. When the resident's mouth is open, places upper denture into the mouth by turning it at an angle. Straightens it. Presses it onto the upper gum line firmly and evenly. Inserts lower denture onto the gum line of the lower jaw. Presses firmly.		
17.	Rinses brush. Cleans, dries, and returns equipment to proper storage. Places basin in designated dirty supply area or returns to storage, depending on facility policy. Drains sink.		
18.	Places used linen in proper container.		
19.	Removes and discards gloves. Washes hands.		
20.	Makes resident comfortable.		
21.	Returns bed to lowest position. Removes privacy measures.		
22.	Leaves call light within resident's reach.		

23.	Washes hands.		
24.	Is courteous and respectful at all times.		
25.	Reports any changes in resident or the appearance of dentures to the nurse. Documents procedure using facility guidelines.		

_____   _____
Date Reviewed   Instructor Signature

_____   _____
Date Performed   Instructor Signature

Providing mouth care for an unconscious resident

		yes	no
1.	Identifies self by name. Identifies resident. Greets resident by name.		
2.	Washes hands.		
3.	Explains procedure to resident. Speaks clearly, slowly, and directly. Maintains face-to-face contact whenever possible.		
4	Provides for resident's privacy with a curtain, screen, or door.		
5.	Adjusts bed to a safe level, usually waist high. Locks bed wheels.		
6.	Puts on gloves.		
7.	Turns resident on his side. Places a towel under his cheek and chin. Places an emesis basin next to the cheek and chin for excess fluid.		
8.	Opens mouth with tongue depressor or by using gentle pressure on the chin. Does not use fingers to open the mouth or keep it open.		
9.	Dips swab in cleaning solution. Squeezes excess solution to prevent aspiration. Wipes inner, outer, and chewing surfaces of the upper and lower teeth, gums, tongue, and inside surfaces of mouth. Changes swab often. Repeats until the mouth is clean.		

10.	Rinses with clean swab dipped in water. Squeezes swab first to remove excess water.		
11.	Removes towel and basin. Pats lips or face dry. Applies lip moisturizer.		
12.	Discards disposable supplies. Places basin in designated dirty supply area or returns to storage, depending on facility policy.		
13.	Places used linen in the proper container.		
14.	Removes and discards gloves. Washes hands.		
15.	Makes resident comfortable.		
16.	Returns bed to lowest position. Removes privacy measures.		
17.	Leaves call light within resident's reach.		
18.	Washes hands.		
19.	Is courteous and respectful at all times.		
20.	Reports any changes in resident to the nurse. Reports any problems with teeth, mouth, tongue, or lips to nurse. These include odor, cracking, sores, bleeding, and any discoloration. Documents procedure using facility guidelines.		

_____   _____
Date Reviewed   Instructor Signature

_____   _____
Date Performed   Instructor Signature

Shaving a resident

		yes	no
1.	Identifies self by name. Identifies resident. Greets resident by name.		
2.	Washes hands.		
3.	Explains procedure to resident. Speaks clearly, slowly, and directly. Maintains face-to-face contact whenever possible.		
4.	Provides for resident's privacy with a curtain, screen, or door.		

Name: _____

5.	Adjusts bed to a safe level, usually waist high. Locks bed wheels.		
6.	Raises head of bed so resident is sitting upright. Places towel across the resident's chest, under his chin.		
7.	Puts on gloves.		
	Shaving using a safety or disposable razor:		
8.	Softens beard with a warm, wet washcloth on the face for a few minutes before shaving. Lathers the face with shaving cream or soap and warm water.		
9.	Holds skin taut. Shaves in direction of the hair growth. Shaves beard in short, downward, and even strokes on face and upward strokes on neck. Rinses the blade often in warm water to keep it clean and wet.		
10.	When finished, washes, rinses, and dries resident's face with a warm, wet washcloth. Offers mirror to resident.		
	Shaving using an electric razor:		
8.	Uses a small brush to clean razor if necessary. Does not use an electric razor near any water source or when oxygen is in use.		
9.	Turns on the razor and holds skin taut. Shaves with smooth, even movements. Shaves beard with back and forth motion in direction of beard growth with foil shaver. Shaves beard in circular motion with three-head shaver. Shaves the chin and under the chin.		
10.	Offers mirror to resident.		
	Final steps:		
11.	Applies aftershave lotion as resident wishes.		
12.	Removes towel and places towel and washcloth in proper container.		

13.	Cleans equipment and stores it. **For safety razor**: rinses razor and stores it. **For disposable razor**: disposes of it in a sharps container. Does not recap razor. **For electric razor**: cleans head of razor. Removes whiskers from razor. Recaps shaving head. Returns razor to case.		
14.	Removes and discards gloves. Washes hands.		
15.	Makes sure that there are no loose hairs. Makes resident comfortable.		
16.	Returns bed to lowest position. Removes privacy measures.		
17.	Leaves call light within resident's reach.		
18.	Washes hands.		
19.	Is courteous and respectful at all times.		
20.	Reports any changes in resident to the nurse. Documents procedure using facility guidelines.		

_____   _____
Date Reviewed   Instructor Signature

_____   _____
Date Performed   Instructor Signature

Providing fingernail care

		yes	no
1.	Identifies self by name. Identifies resident. Greets resident by name.		
2.	Washes hands.		
3.	Explains procedure to resident. Speaks clearly, slowly, and directly. Maintains face-to-face contact whenever possible.		
4.	Provides for resident's privacy with a curtain, screen, or door.		
5.	If the resident is in bed, adjusts bed to safe working level, usually waist high. Locks bed wheels.		

6.	Fills basin halfway with warm water. Tests water temperature with thermometer or wrist. Ensures it is safe. Has resident check water temperature. Adjusts if necessary. Places basin at a comfortable level for resident.		
7.	Puts on gloves.		
8.	Soaks resident's nails in the basin of water. Soaks all 10 fingertips for at 5–10 minutes.		
9.	Removes hands from basin. Washes hands with soapy washcloth. Rinses. Pats hands dry with towel, including between fingers. Removes hand basin.		
10.	Places resident's hands on the towel. Gently cleans under each fingernail with orangewood stick.		
11.	Wipes orangewood stick on towel after each nail. Washes resident's hands again. Dries them thoroughly, especially between fingers.		
12.	Shapes nails with file or emery board. Files in a curve. Finishes with nails smooth and free of rough edges.		
13.	Applies lotion from fingertips to wrists. Removes excess lotion with a towel.		
14.	Empties, rinses, and wipes basin. Places basin in designated dirty supply area or returns to storage, depending on facility policy.		
15.	Places used linen in the proper container.		
16.	Removes and discards gloves. Washes hands.		
17.	Makes resident comfortable.		
18.	Returns bed to lowest position. Removes privacy measures.		
19.	Leaves call light within resident's reach.		

20.	Washes hands.		
21.	Is courteous and respectful at all times.		
22.	Reports any changes in resident to the nurse. Documents procedure using facility guidelines.		

_____   _____
Date Reviewed   Instructor Signature

_____   _____
Date Performed   Instructor Signature

Combing or brushing hair

		yes	no
	Uses hair care products that the resident prefers for his or her type of hair.		
1.	Identifies self by name. Identifies resident. Greets resident by name.		
2.	Washes hands.		
3.	Explains procedure to resident. Speaks clearly, slowly, and directly. Maintains face-to-face contact whenever possible.		
4.	Provides for resident's privacy with a curtain, screen, or door.		
5.	If the resident is in bed, adjusts bed to safe working level, usually waist high. Raises head of bed so resident is sitting upright. Locks bed wheels.		
6.	Places towel under head or around shoulders.		
7.	Removes any hair pins, hair ties, and clips.		
8.	Removes tangles first by dividing hair into small sections. Holds lock of hair just above tangle so hair is not pulled at the scalp. Combs through tangles.		
9.	After tangles are removed, brushes two-inch sections of hair at a time.		
10.	Neatly styles hair as resident prefers. Avoids childish hairstyles. Offers mirror to resident.		

Name: _____

		yes	no
11.	Makes resident comfortable.		
12.	Returns bed to lowest position. Removes privacy measures.		
13.	Returns supplies to proper storage. Cleans hair from comb or brush. Cleans comb and brush.		
14.	Places used linen in the proper container.		
15.	Leaves call light within resident's reach.		
16.	Washes hands.		
17.	Is courteous and respectful at all times.		
18.	Reports any changes in resident to the nurse. Documents procedure using facility guidelines.		

_____ _____
Date Reviewed   Instructor Signature

_____ _____
Date Performed   Instructor Signature

Dressing a resident

		yes	no
	When putting on all items, moves resident's body gently and naturally. Avoids force and overextension of limbs and joints.		
1.	Identifies self by name. Identifies resident. Greets resident by name.		
2.	Washes hands.		
3.	Explains procedure to resident. Speaks clearly, slowly, and directly. Maintains face-to-face contact whenever possible.		
4.	Provides for resident's privacy with a curtain, screen, or door.		
5.	Asks resident what she would like to wear. Dresses her in outfit of choice.		
6.	After placing bath blanket, removes gown or top without exposing resident. Takes clothes off stronger side first when undressing. Then removes from weaker side. Places gown or top in proper container for cleaning.		
7.	Helps resident slide top over the head. Inserts weaker arm through sleeve first, then the stronger arm. Helps resident lean forward to smooth down top. If the top fastens in the front, slides hand through one sleeve and grasps resident's hand on the weaker side, pulling it through. Helps resident lean forward and arranges the top across the back. Pulls the second sleeve onto the stronger side and fastens the top.		
8.	Helps resident to put on skirt or pants. Puts weaker leg through skirt or pants first. Raises buttocks or turns resident from side to side to draw pants over the buttocks up to waist. Fastens pants or skirt.		
9.	Rolls one sock over weaker foot. Makes sure heel is in heel of sock. Smoothes over foot to remove wrinkles. Repeats for other foot.		
10.	Places bed at the lowest position. Locks bed wheels. Helps resident into sitting position. Puts on nonskid footwear, weaker foot first. Fastens securely.		
11.	Finishes with resident dressed appropriately. Makes sure clothing is right-side out and zippers/buttons are fastened.		
12.	Makes resident comfortable. Leaves bed in lowest position. Removes privacy measures.		
13.	Leaves call light within resident's reach.		

14.	Washes hands.		
15.	Is courteous and respectful at all times.		
16.	Reports any changes in resident to the nurse. Documents procedure using facility guidelines.		

_____ _____
Date Reviewed   Instructor Signature

_____ _____
Date Performed   Instructor Signature

13
Vital Signs

Measuring and recording oral temperature		yes	no
	Does not take an oral temperature on a resident who has smoked, eaten or drunk fluids, chewed gum, or exercised within the last 10 to 20 minutes.		
1.	Identifies self by name. Identifies resident. Greets resident by name.		
2.	Washes hands.		
3.	Explains procedure to resident. Speaks clearly, slowly, and directly. Maintains face-to-face contact whenever possible.		
4.	Provides for resident's privacy with a curtain, screen, or door.		
5.	Puts on gloves.		
6.	*Digital thermometer*: Puts on disposable sheath. Turns on thermometer. Waits until *ready* sign appears.		
	Electronic thermometer: Removes probe from base unit. Puts on probe cover.		
	Mercury-free thermometer: Holds thermometer by stem. Before inserting thermometer in resident's mouth, shakes thermometer down to below the lowest number (at least below 96°F or 35°C).		
7.	*Digital thermometer*: Inserts end of digital thermometer into resident's mouth. Places under tongue and to one side.		
	Electronic thermometer: Inserts the covered probe into resident's mouth. Places under tongue and to one side.		
	Mercury-free thermometer: Puts on disposable sheath if available. Gently inserts bulb end of thermometer into resident's mouth. Places under tongue and to one side.		
8.	*For all thermometers*: Tells resident to hold thermometer in his mouth with his lips closed. Assists as necessary. Asks resident not to bite down or to talk.		
	Digital thermometer: Holds in place until thermometer blinks or beeps.		
	Electronic thermometer: Holds in place until a tone is heard or a flashing or steady light is seen.		
	Mercury-free thermometer: Leaves thermometer in place for at least three minutes.		
9.	*Digital thermometer*: Removes thermometer. Reads temperature on display screen. Remembers temperature reading.		
	Electronic thermometer: Reads temperature on the display screen. Remembers temperature reading. Removes probe.		
	Mercury-free thermometer: Removes thermometer. Wipes with tissue from stem to bulb or removes sheath. Disposes of tissue or sheath. Holds thermometer at eye level. Rotates until line appears, rolling the thermometer between thumb and forefinger. Reads temperature. Remembers temperature reading.		

Name: _____

10.	**Digital thermometer**: Using a tissue, removes and discards sheath. Cleans thermometer according to policy. Replaces thermometer in case.		
	Electronic thermometer: Presses eject button to discard the cover. Returns probe to the holder.		
	Mercury-free thermometer: Cleans thermometer according to policy. Rinses with clean water. Returns it to case or container.		
11.	Removes and discards gloves. Washes hands.		
12.	Immediately records temperature, date, time, and method used (oral).		
13.	Makes resident comfortable. Removes privacy measures.		
14.	Leaves call light within resident's reach.		
15.	Washes hands.		
16.	Is courteous and respectful at all times.		
17.	Reports any changes in resident to the nurse.		

_____   _____
Date Reviewed   Instructor Signature

_____   _____
Date Performed   Instructor Signature

Measuring and recording rectal temperature

		yes	no
1.	Identifies self by name. Identifies resident. Greets resident by name.		
2.	Washes hands.		
3.	Explains procedure to resident. Speaks clearly, slowly, and directly. Maintains face-to-face contact whenever possible.		
4.	Provides for resident's privacy with a curtain, screen, or door.		
5.	Adjusts bed to a safe level, usually waist high. Locks bed wheels.		
6.	Helps resident to left-lying (Sims') position.		
7.	Folds back linens to expose only rectal area.		
8.	Puts on gloves.		
9.	**Digital thermometer**: Puts on disposable sheath. Turns on thermometer. Waits until _ready_ sign appears.		
	Electronic thermometer: Removes probe from base unit. Puts on probe cover.		
	Mercury-free thermometer: Holds thermometer by stem. Shakes thermometer down to below the lowest number. Puts on disposable sheath.		
10.	Applies a small amount of lubricant to tip of bulb or probe cover (or applies prelubricated cover).		
11.	Separates the buttocks. Gently inserts thermometer one-half to one inch into rectum. Stops if resistance is met. Does not force thermometer into rectum.		
12.	Replaces sheet over buttocks while holding on to thermometer at all times.		
13.	**Digital thermometer**: Holds thermometer in place until thermometer blinks or beeps.		
	Electronic thermometer: Holds in place until a tone is heard or a flashing or steady light is seen.		
	Mercury-free thermometer: Holds thermometer in place for at least three minutes.		
14.	Gently removes thermometer. Wipes with tissue from stem to bulb or removes sheath or cover. Discards tissue or sheath.		
15.	Reads thermometer at eye level. Remembers temperature reading.		

Name: _____

16.	**Digital thermometer**: Cleans thermometer according to policy. Replaces thermometer in case.		
	Electronic thermometer: Presses eject button to discard the cover. Returns probe to holder.		
	Mercury-free thermometer: Cleans thermometer according to policy. Rinses with clean water. Returns it to case or container.		
17.	Removes and discards gloves.		
18.	Washes hands.		
19.	Makes resident comfortable.		
20.	Immediately records temperature, date, time, and method used (rectal).		
21.	Returns bed to lowest position. Removes privacy measures.		
22.	Leaves call light within resident's reach.		
23.	Washes hands.		
24.	Is courteous and respectful at all times.		
25.	Reports any changes in resident to the nurse.		

_____   _____
Date Reviewed   Instructor Signature

_____   _____
Date Performed   Instructor Signature

Measuring and recording tympanic temperature

		yes	no
1.	Identifies self by name. Identifies resident. Greets resident by name.		
2.	Washes hands.		
3.	Explains procedure to resident. Speaks clearly, slowly, and directly. Maintains face-to-face contact whenever possible.		
4.	Provides for resident's privacy with a curtain, screen, or door.		
5.	Puts on gloves.		
6.	Puts a disposable sheath over earpiece of the thermometer.		
7.	Positions resident's head so that the ear is in front of self. Straightens ear canal by gently pulling up and back on the outside edge of the ear. Inserts covered probe into the ear canal. Presses button.		
8.	Holds thermometer in place until thermometer blinks or beeps.		
9.	Reads temperature. Remembers temperature reading.		
10.	Disposes of sheath. Returns thermometer to storage or to the battery charger if thermometer is rechargeable.		
11.	Removes and discards gloves. Washes hands.		
12.	Immediately records temperature, date, time, and method used (tympanic).		
13.	Makes resident comfortable. Removes privacy measures.		
14.	Leaves call light within resident's reach.		
15.	Washes hands.		
16.	Is courteous and respectful at all times.		
17.	Reports any changes in resident to the nurse.		

_____   _____
Date Reviewed   Instructor Signature

_____   _____
Date Performed   Instructor Signature

Measuring and recording axillary temperature

		yes	no
1.	Identifies self by name. Identifies resident. Greets resident by name.		
2.	Washes hands.		
3.	Explains procedure to resident. Speaks clearly, slowly, and directly. Maintains face-to-face contact whenever possible.		

4.	Provides for resident's privacy with a curtain, screen, or door.		
5.	Adjusts bed to a safe level, usually waist high. Locks bed wheels.		
6.	Puts on gloves.		
7.	Removes resident's arm from sleeve of gown. Wipes axillary area with tissues.		
8.	*Digital thermometer*: Puts on disposable sheath. Turns on thermometer. Waits until *ready* sign appears.		
	Electronic thermometer: Removes probe from base unit. Puts on probe cover.		
	Mercury-free thermometer: Holds thermometer by stem. Shakes thermometer down to below the lowest number. Puts on disposable sheath.		
9.	Positions thermometer (bulb end for mercury-free) in center of the armpit. Folds resident's arm over chest.		
10.	*Digital thermometer*: Holds thermometer in place until thermometer blinks or beeps.		
	Electronic thermometer: Holds in place until a tone is heard or a flashing or steady light is seen.		
	Mercury-free thermometer: Holds thermometer in place, with the arm close against the side, for eight to ten minutes.		
11.	*Digital thermometer*: Removes thermometer. Reads temperature on display screen. Remembers temperature reading.		
	Electronic thermometer: Reads temperature on the display screen. Remembers temperature reading. Removes probe.		

	Mercury-free thermometer: Removes thermometer. Wipes with tissue from stem to bulb or removes sheath. Disposes of tissue or sheath. Reads temperature. Remembers temperature reading.		
12.	*Digital thermometer*: Using a tissue, removes and discards sheath. Cleans thermometer according to policy. Replaces thermometer in case.		
	Electronic thermometer: Presses eject button to discard the cover. Returns probe to the holder.		
	Mercury-free thermometer: Cleans thermometer according to policy. Rinses with clean water. Returns it to case or container.		
13.	Removes and discards gloves. Washes hands.		
14.	Puts resident's arm back into sleeve of gown. Makes resident comfortable.		
15.	Immediately records temperature, date, time, and method used (axillary).		
16.	Returns bed to lowest position. Removes privacy measures.		
17.	Leaves call light within resident's reach.		
18.	Washes hands.		
19.	Is courteous and respectful at all times.		
20.	Reports any changes in resident to the nurse.		

_____   _____
Date Reviewed   Instructor Signature

_____   _____
Date Performed   Instructor Signature

Counting and recording radial pulse and counting and recording respirations

		yes	no
1.	Identifies self by name. Identifies resident. Greets resident by name.		
2.	Washes hands.		
3.	Explains procedure to resident. Speaks clearly, slowly, and directly. Maintains face-to-face contact whenever possible.		
4.	Provides for resident's privacy with a curtain, screen, or door.		
5.	Places fingertips of index finger and middle finger on the thumb side of resident's wrist to locate radial pulse. Does not use thumb.		
6.	Counts beats for one full minute.		
7.	Keeps fingertips on resident's wrist. Counts respirations for one full minute. Observes for pattern and character of resident's breathing.		
8.	Washes hands.		
9.	Records pulse rate, date, time, and method used (radial). Records respiratory rate and pattern or character of breathing.		
10.	Removes privacy measures. Makes resident comfortable.		
11.	Leaves call light within resident's reach.		
12.	Washes hands.		
13.	Is courteous and respectful at all times.		
14.	Reports any changes in resident to the nurse.		

_____ _____
Date Reviewed   Instructor Signature

_____ _____
Date Performed   Instructor Signature

Counting and recording apical pulse

		yes	no
1.	Identifies self by name. Identifies resident. Greets resident by name.		
2.	Washes hands.		
3.	Explains procedure to resident. Speaks clearly, slowly, and directly. Maintains face-to-face contact whenever possible.		
4.	Provides for resident's privacy with a curtain, screen, or door.		
5.	Before using stethoscope, wipes diaphragm and earpieces with alcohol wipes.		
6.	Fits earpieces of the stethoscope snugly in ears. Places flat metal diaphragm on the left side of the chest, just below the nipple. Listens for the heartbeat.		
7.	Counts beats for one full minute. Leaves stethoscope in place to count respirations.		
8.	Records pulse rate, date, time, and method used (apical). Notes any irregularities in the rhythm.		
9.	Cleans earpieces and diaphragm of stethoscope with alcohol wipes.		
10.	Makes resident comfortable. Removes privacy measures.		
11.	Leaves call light within resident's reach.		
12.	Washes hands.		
13.	Is courteous and respectful at all times.		
14.	Reports any changes in resident to the nurse.		

_____ _____
Date Reviewed   Instructor Signature

_____ _____
Date Performed   Instructor Signature

Counting and recording apical-radial pulse

		yes	no
	Finds coworker to assist.		
1.	Identifies self by name. Identifies resident. Greets resident by name.		
2.	Washes hands.		
3.	Explains procedure to resident. Speaks clearly, slowly, and directly. Maintains face-to-face contact whenever possible.		
4.	Provides for resident's privacy with a curtain, screen, or door.		
5.	Before using stethoscope, wipes diaphragm and earpieces with alcohol wipes.		
6.	Fits earpieces of stethoscope snugly in ears. Places flat metal diaphragm on the left side of the chest, just below the nipple. Listens for the heartbeat.		
7.	Coworker places her fingertips on the thumb side of resident's wrist to locate the radial pulse.		
8.	After both pulses have been located, looks at the second hand of watch. When the second hand reaches the "12" or "6," says, "Start," and both people count beats for one full minute. Says, "Stop" after one minute.		
9.	Records both pulse rates, date, time, and method used (apical-radial). Records pulse deficit if the pulse rates are not the same. Notes any irregularities in the pulse rhythm.		
10.	Cleans earpieces and diaphragm of stethoscope with alcohol wipes.		
11.	Makes resident comfortable. Removes privacy measures.		
12.	Leaves call light within resident's reach.		
13.	Washes hands.		
14.	Is courteous and respectful at all times.		
15.	Reports any changes in resident to the nurse.		

_____   _____
Date Reviewed   Instructor Signature

_____   _____
Date Performed   Instructor Signature

Measuring and recording blood pressure manually

		yes	no
1.	Identifies self by name. Identifies resident. Greets resident by name.		
2.	Washes hands.		
3.	Explains procedure to resident. Speaks clearly, slowly, and directly. Maintains face-to-face contact whenever possible.		
4.	Provides for resident's privacy with a curtain, screen, or door.		
5.	Before using the stethoscope, wipes diaphragm and earpieces with alcohol wipes.		
6.	Asks resident to roll up his or her sleeve, approximately five inches above the elbow. Does not measure blood pressure over clothing.		
7.	Positions resident's arm with palm up, with arm level with the heart.		
8.	With the valve open, squeezes the cuff. Makes sure it is completely deflated.		
9.	Places blood pressure cuff snugly on resident's upper arm. Makes sure center of the cuff with sensor/arrow is placed over the brachial artery (1-1½ inches above the elbow, toward inside of elbow).		
10.	Asks resident to remain still and quiet.		
11.	Locates brachial pulse with fingertips.		

12.	Places earpieces of the stethoscope in ears.		
13.	Places diaphragm of the stethoscope over brachial artery.		
14.	Closes the valve (clockwise) until it stops. Does not over-tighten it.		
15.	Inflates cuff to between 160 mm Hg to 180 mm Hg. If a beat is heard immediately upon cuff deflation, completely deflates cuff. Reinflates cuff to no more than 200 mm Hg.		
16.	Opens valve slightly with thumb and index finger. Deflates cuff slowly.		
17.	Watches gauge. Listens for sound of pulse.		
18.	Remembers reading at which the first clear pulse sound is heard. This is the systolic pressure.		
19.	Continues listening for a change or muffling of pulse sound. The point of a change or the point the sound disappears is the diastolic pressure. Remembers this reading.		
20.	Opens the valve. Deflates cuff completely. Removes cuff.		
21.	Washes hands.		
22.	Records both the systolic and diastolic pressures. Records numbers like a fraction, with the systolic reading on top and the diastolic reading on the bottom (for example: 119/79). Notes which arm was used. Uses *RA* for right arm and *LA* for left arm.		
23.	Wipes diaphragm and earpieces of the stethoscope with alcohol. Stores equipment.		
24.	Makes resident comfortable. Removes privacy measures.		
25.	Leaves call light within resident's reach.		

26.	Washes hands.		
27.	Is courteous and respectful at all times.		
28.	Reports any changes in resident to the nurse.		

Date Reviewed _____ Instructor Signature

Date Performed _____ Instructor Signature

Measuring and recording blood pressure electronically

		yes	no
1.	Identifies self by name. Identifies resident. Greets resident by name.		
2.	Washes hands.		
3.	Explains procedure to resident. Speaks clearly, slowly, and directly. Maintains face-to-face contact whenever possible.		
4.	Provides for resident's privacy with a curtain, screen, or door.		
5.	Asks resident to roll up his or her sleeve, approximately five inches above the elbow. Does not measure blood pressure over clothing.		
6.	Positions resident's arm with palm up, with arm level with the heart.		
7.	Places blood pressure cuff snugly on resident's upper arm. Makes sure center of the cuff with sensor/arrow is placed over the brachial artery (1-1½ inches above the elbow, toward inside of elbow).		
8.	Asks resident to remain still and quiet.		
9.	Turns on blood pressure machine. Presses start.		
10.	Waits for machine to complete measurement and for cuff to deflate.		
11.	Removes cuff.		

12.	Washes hands.		
13.	Records both the systolic and diastolic pressures. Notes which arm was used.		
14.	Makes resident comfortable. Removes privacy measures.		
15.	Leaves call light within resident's reach.		
16.	Washes hands.		
17.	Is courteous and respectful at all times.		
18.	Reports any changes in resident to the nurse.		

_____   _____
Date Reviewed   Instructor Signature

_____   _____
Date Performed   Instructor Signature

14
Nutrition and Fluid Balance

Feeding a resident			
		yes	no
1.	Identifies self by name. Identifies resident. Greets resident by name.		
2.	Washes hands.		
3.	Explains procedure to resident. Speaks clearly, slowly, and directly. Maintains face-to-face contact whenever possible.		
4.	Provides for resident's privacy with a curtain, screen, or door.		
5.	Looks at diet card or menu. Asks resident to state his name. Verifies that resident has received the right tray.		
6.	Raises head of the bed. Makes sure resident is in an upright sitting position (at a 90-degree angle).		
7.	Adjusts bed height so that caregiver is at resident's eye level. Locks bed wheels.		

8.	Places meal tray where it can be easily seen by the resident, such as on the overbed table.		
9.	Helps resident to clean hands with hand wipes if resident cannot do it on her own.		
10.	Helps resident to put on clothing protector if desired.		
11.	Sits facing resident. Sits at resident's eye level. Sits on the stronger side if resident has one-sided weakness.		
12.	Tells resident what foods are on plate. Offers a drink of beverage and asks what resident would like to eat first.		
13.	Offers food in bite-sized pieces, telling the resident the content of each bite of food offered. Alternates types of food, allowing for resident's preferences. Does not feed all of one type before offering another type. Makes sure resident's mouth is empty before the next bite or sip is offered. Reports any swallowing problems to the nurse immediately. If resident has one-sided weakness, directs food to the stronger side.		
14.	Offers sips of beverage to resident throughout the meal.		
15.	Talks with resident during the meal.		
16.	Uses washcloths or wipes to wipe food from resident's mouth and hands as needed during the meal. Wipes again at the end of the meal.		
17.	Removes clothing protector if used. Disposes of it and used washcloths or wipes in proper container.		

18.	Removes food tray. Checks for eyeglasses, dentures, hearing aids, or any personal items before removing tray. Places tray in proper area to be picked up.		
19.	Makes resident comfortable. Keeps resident in the upright position for at least 30 minutes after eating and drinking if ordered. Makes sure the bed is free from crumbs.		
20.	Returns bed to lowest position. Removes privacy measures.		
21.	Leaves call light within resident's reach.		
22.	Washes hands.		
23.	Is courteous and respectful at all times.		
24.	Reports any changes in resident to the nurse. Documents procedure using facility guidelines. Records intake of solid food and fluids properly.		

Date Reviewed   Instructor Signature

Date Performed   Instructor Signature

Measuring and recording intake and output

		yes	no
	Measures intake first.		
1.	Identifies self by name. Identifies resident. Greets resident by name.		
2.	Washes hands.		
3.	Explains procedure to resident. Speaks clearly, slowly, and directly. Maintains face-to-face contact whenever possible.		
4.	Provides for resident's privacy with a curtain, screen, or door.		
5.	Notes amount of fluid resident is served on paper.		
6.	When the resident has finished a meal or snack, measures any leftover fluids. Notes this amount on paper.		

7.	Subtracts leftover amount from the amount served. Converts from ounces to milliliters (mL) by multiplying by 30.		
8.	Records amount of fluid consumed (in mL) in input column on I&O sheet. Records time and what fluid was consumed.		
9.	Washes hands.		
	Measures output.		
1.	Washes hands.		
2.	Puts on gloves before handling bedpan/urinal.		
3.	Pours contents of the bedpan or urinal into graduate. Does not spill or splash any of the urine.		
4.	Places graduate on flat surface. Measures amount of urine at eye level. Keeps container level.		
5.	After measuring urine, empties contents of graduate into toilet without splashing. Rinses graduate and pours rinse water into the toilet. Rinses bedpan/urinal and pours rinse water into the toilet. Flushes the toilet.		
6.	Places graduate and bedpan in area for cleaning or cleans and stores according to policy.		
7.	Removes and discards gloves.		
8.	Washes hands before recording output.		
9.	Records time and amount of urine in output column on sheet. Reports any changes to the nurse.		

Date Reviewed   Instructor Signature

Date Performed   Instructor Signature

Serving fresh water

		yes	no
1.	Identifies self by name. Identifies resident. Greets resident by name.		

Name: _____

		yes	no
2.	Washes hands.		
3.	Puts on gloves.		
4.	Scoops ice into the water pitcher, without touching ice scoop to pitcher. Adds fresh water, without allowing pitcher to touch the faucet.		
5.	Uses and stores ice scoop properly. Places scoop into the proper receptacle after each use.		
6.	Takes pitcher to resident.		
7.	Pours water into the cup for the resident. Offers resident a drink of water. Leaves pitcher and cup at the bedside.		
8.	Makes sure pitcher and cup are light enough for the resident to lift. Leaves a straw if resident desires it and is allowed to use one.		
9.	Makes resident comfortable.		
10.	Leaves call light within resident's reach.		
11.	Removes and discards gloves. Washes hands.		
12.	Is courteous and respectful at all times.		

_____   _____
Date Reviewed   Instructor Signature

_____   _____
Date Performed   Instructor Signature

15
The Gastrointestinal System

Assisting a resident with use of a bedpan			
		yes	no
1.	Identifies self by name. Identifies resident. Greets resident by name.		
2.	Washes hands.		
3.	Explains procedure to resident. Speaks clearly, slowly, and directly. Maintains face-to-face contact whenever possible.		
4.	Provides for resident's privacy with a curtain, screen, or door.		
5.	Adjusts bed to safe level, usually waist high. Raises the far bed rail. Before placing bedpan, lowers head of bed. Locks bed wheels.		
6.	Puts on gloves.		
7.	Covers resident with a bath blanket. Asks him to hold it while pulling down the top covers underneath. Does not expose more of resident than is needed.		
8.	Places bed protector under resident's buttocks and hips.		
9.	Asks resident to remove undergarments or helps him do so.		
10.	Places bedpan near his hips in correct position. **Standard bedpan** should be positioned with the wider end aligned with resident's buttocks. **Fracture pan** should be positioned with handle toward foot of bed.		
11.	If resident is able, asks him to raise hips by pushing with feet and hands on the count of three. Slides bedpan under his hips.		
	If a resident cannot help in any way, keeps bed flat and rolls resident away from self, toward raised bed rail. Slips bedpan under the hips and rolls him back onto bedpan. Keeps bedpan centered underneath.		
12.	Removes and discards gloves. Washes hands.		
13.	Raises head of the bed until resident is in a sitting position. Props resident into a semi-sitting position using pillows. Makes sure both bed rails are up and bed is in its lowest position.		

14.	Places toilet paper and wipes within resident's reach. Asks resident to clean his hands with a hand wipe when finished if he is able.		
15.	Leaves call light within resident's reach. Washes hands. Asks resident to signal when finished. Leaves room and closes the door.		
16.	When called by the resident, returns and washes hands. Puts on clean gloves.		
17.	Raises bed to safe level. Lowers head of the bed. Makes sure resident is still covered. Does not overexpose resident. Lowers near bed rail.		
18.	Removes bedpan carefully. Covers bedpan.		
19.	Gives perineal care if help is needed. Wipes from front to back. Dries perineal area with a towel. Removes bed protector. Helps resident put on under garment. Covers resident and removes bath blanket.		
20.	Places towel and bath blanket in a hamper or bag, and discards disposable supplies.		
21.	Takes bedpan to the bathroom. Notes color, odor, amount, and consistency of contents. Empties contents into toilet unless the nurse needs to check the contents. Does not discard it if anything unusual about the stool or urine is noted.		
22.	Turns the faucet on with a paper towel. Rinses the bedpan with cold water and empties it into the toilet. Flushes toilet. Places bedpan in area for cleaning or cleans and stores it according to policy.		

23.	Removes and discards gloves. Washes hands.		
24.	Makes resident comfortable.		
25.	Returns bed to lowest position. Removes privacy measures.		
26.	Leaves call light within resident's reach.		
27.	Washes hands.		
28.	Is courteous and respectful at all times.		
29.	Reports any changes in resident to the nurse. Documents procedure using facility guidelines.		

_____   _____
Date Reviewed   Instructor Signature

_____   _____
Date Performed   Instructor Signature

Assisting a male resident with a urinal

		yes	no
1.	Identifies self by name. Identifies resident. Greets resident by name.		
2.	Washes hands.		
3.	Explains procedure to resident. Speaks clearly, slowly, and directly. Maintains face-to-face contact whenever possible.		
4.	Provides for resident's privacy with a curtain, screen, or door.		
5.	Adjusts bed to a safe level, usually waist high. Locks bed wheels.		
6.	Puts on gloves.		
7.	Places bed protector under the resident's buttocks and hips.		
8.	Hands urinal to the resident. If the resident cannot do so himself, places urinal between his legs and positions penis inside the urinal. Replaces bed covers.		
9.	Removes and discards gloves. Washes hands.		

10.	Raises the head of the bed. Makes sure both bed rails are up and bed is in its lowest position. Places wipes within resident's reach. Asks resident to clean his hands with a hand wipe when finished if he is able. Leaves call light within reach. Washes hands. Asks resident to signal when done. Leaves room and closes the door.		
11.	When called by the resident, returns and washes hands. Puts on clean gloves.		
12.	Removes urinal. Removes bed protector. Discards disposable supplies.		
13.	Takes urinal to the bathroom. Notes color, odor, amount, and qualities of contents before flushing. Empties contents into toilet unless the nurse needs to check the contents.		
14.	Turns the faucet on with a paper towel. Rinses the urinal with cold water and empties rinse water into the toilet. Flushes toilet. Places urinal in proper area for cleaning or cleans and stores it according to policy.		
15.	Removes and discards gloves. Washes hands.		
16.	Returns bed to lowest position. Removes privacy measures.		
17.	Makes resident comfortable.		
18.	Leaves call light within resident's reach.		
19.	Washes hands.		
20.	Is courteous and respectful at all times.		
21.	Reports any changes in resident to the nurse. Documents procedure using facility guidelines.		

_____ _____
Date Reviewed   Instructor Signature

_____ _____
Date Performed   Instructor Signature

Helping a resident use a portable commode

		yes	no
1.	Identifies self by name. Identifies resident. Greets resident by name.		
2.	Washes hands.		
3.	Explains procedure to resident. Speaks clearly, slowly, and directly. Maintains face-to-face contact whenever possible.		
4.	Provides for resident's privacy with a curtain, screen, or door.		
5.	Locks commode wheels. Adjusts bed to lowest position. Locks bed wheels.		
6.	Puts on gloves.		
7.	Helps resident out of bed and to portable commode. Makes sure resident is wearing nonskid footwear that is securely fastened.		
8.	If needed, helps resident remove clothing and sit comfortably on toilet seat. Places blanket over resident's legs. Places toilet paper and wipes within resident's reach. Asks resident to clean his hands with a hand wipe when finished if he is able.		
9.	Leaves call light within resident's reach. Removes and discards gloves. Washes hands. Asks resident to signal when finished. Leaves room and closes the door.		
10.	When called by the resident, returns and washes hands. Puts on clean gloves.		
11.	Gives perineal care if help is needed. Wipes from front to back. Dries perineal area with a towel. Helps resident put on undergarment. Places towel in a hamper or bag. Discards disposable supplies.		
12.	Removes and discards gloves. Washes hands.		

13.	Helps resident back to bed. Leaves bed in lowest position. Removes privacy measures.		
14.	Makes resident comfortable.		
15.	Puts on clean gloves.		
16.	Removes waste basin. Notes color, odor, amount, and consistency of contents. Empties contents into toilet unless nurse needs to check the contents.		
17.	Turns the faucet on with a paper towel. Rinses the container with cold water and empties it into the toilet. Flushes toilet. Places container in proper area for cleaning or cleans it according to facility policy.		
18.	Removes and discards gloves. Washes hands.		
19.	Leaves call light within resident's reach.		
20.	Washes hands.		
21.	Is courteous and respectful at all times.		
22.	Reports any changes in resident to the nurse. Documents procedure using facility guidelines.		

_____ _____
Date Reviewed   Instructor Signature

_____ _____
Date Performed   Instructor Signature

Giving a cleansing enema

		yes	no
1.	Identifies self by name. Identifies resident. Greets resident by name.		
2.	Washes hands.		
3.	Explains procedure to resident. Speaks clearly, slowly, and directly. Maintains face-to-face contact whenever possible.		
4.	Provides for resident's privacy with a curtain, screen, or door.		
5.	Adjusts bed to a safe level, usually waist high. Locks bed wheels.		

6.	Puts on gloves.		
7.	Places bed protector under resident. Asks resident to remove undergarments or helps him do so.		
8.	Helps resident into left-sided Sims' position. Places bedpan close to resident's body. Covers with a bath blanket.		
9.	Places IV pole beside the bed.		
10.	Clamps enema tube. Prepares the enema solution. Adds specific additive if ordered. Fills bag with 500 to 1000 mL of warm water and swishes fluid to mix well. Checks water temperature with bath thermometer.		
11.	Unclamps tube. Lets a small amount of solution run through the tubing to release the air. Reclamps tube.		
12.	Hangs bag on IV pole. Using the tape measure, makes sure bottom of enema bag is not more than 12 inches above resident's anus.		
13.	Uncovers only enough to expose the resident's anus. Lubricates 2–4 inches of the tip of the tubing with lubricating jelly.		
14.	Asks resident to breathe deeply.		
15.	Places one hand on upper buttock. Lifts to expose the anus. Asks resident to take a deep breath and exhale. Using other hand, inserts tip of the tubing 2–4 inches into the rectum. Stops immediately if resistance is felt or if the resident complains of pain.		
16.	Unclamps tubing. Allows solution to flow slowly into the rectum. Asks resident to take slow, deep breaths. Encourages him to take as much of the solution as possible.		

17.	Clamps tubing before the bag is empty when the solution is almost gone. Removes tip from rectum. Places tip into the enema bag. Does not contaminate self, resident, or bed linens.		
18.	Asks resident to hold the solution inside as long as possible.		
19.	Helps resident to use bedpan or commode, or to get to the bathroom. Raises head of the bed if resident is using bedpan. Makes sure both bed rails are up and bed is in its lowest position. If resident uses a commode or bathroom, puts on robe and nonskid footwear. Lowers the bed to its lowest position before the resident gets up.		
20.	Removes and discards gloves. Washes hands.		
21.	Places toilet paper and wipes within resident's reach. Asks resident to clean his hands with a hand wipe when finished if he is able. If the resident is using the bathroom, asks him not to flush the toilet when finished.		
22.	Places call light within resident's reach. Washes hands. Asks resident to signal when finished. Leaves room and closes the door.		
23.	When called by the resident, returns and washes hands. Puts on clean gloves.		
24.	Raises bed to safe level. Lowers head of bed if raised. Makes sure resident is still covered. Does not overexpose the resident. Lowers bed rail on working side if it was raised.		
25.	Removes bedpan carefully and gently. Covers bedpan.		

26.	Gives perineal care if help is needed. Wipes from front to back. Dries perineal area with a towel. Helps resident put on undergarment. Covers resident and removes the bath blanket.		
27.	Removes and discards bed protector. Places towel in a hamper or bag, and discards disposable supplies.		
28.	Takes bedpan to the bathroom. Calls nurse to observe enema results, whether in bedpan or in toilet. Empties contents into toilet.		
29.	Turns the faucet on with a paper towel. Rinses the bedpan with cold water and empties it into the toilet. Flushes toilet. Places bedpan in proper area for cleaning or cleans and stores it according to policy.		
30.	Removes and discards gloves. Washes hands.		
31.	Makes resident comfortable.		
32.	Returns bed to lowest position. Removes privacy measures.		
33.	Leaves call light within resident's reach.		
34.	Washes hands.		
35.	Is courteous and respectful at all times.		
36.	Reports any changes in resident to the nurse. Documents procedure using facility guidelines.		

_____   _____
Date Reviewed   Instructor Signature

_____   _____
Date Performed   Instructor Signature

Name: _____

Giving a commercial enema		yes	no
1.	Identifies self by name. Identifies resident. Greets resident by name.		
2.	Washes hands.		
3.	Explains procedure to resident. Speaks clearly, slowly, and directly. Maintains face-to-face contact whenever possible.		
4.	Provides for resident's privacy with a curtain, screen, or door.		
5.	Adjusts bed to a safe level, usually waist high. Locks bed wheels.		
6.	Puts on gloves.		
7.	Places bed protector under resident. Asks resident to remove undergarments or helps him do so.		
8.	Helps resident into left-sided Sims' position. Places bedpan close to resident's body. Covers with a bath blanket.		
9.	Uncovers resident enough to expose anus only.		
10.	Adds extra lubricating jelly to the tip of bottle if needed.		
11.	Asks resident to breathe deeply to relieve cramps during procedure.		
12.	Places one hand on the upper buttock. Lifts to expose anus. Asks resident to take a deep breath and exhale. Using other hand, inserts tip of the tubing about 1½ inches into the rectum. Stops immediately if resistance is felt or if the resident complains of pain.		
13.	Slowly squeezes and rolls the enema container so that solution runs inside resident. Stops when container is almost empty.		
14.	Removes tip from rectum, continuing to keep pressure on the container until bottle is placed inside the box upside down.		
15.	Asks resident to hold solution inside as long as possible.		
16.	Helps resident to use bedpan or commode, or to go to the bathroom. Raises head of bed if resident is using bedpan. Makes sure both bed rails are up and bed is in its lowest position. If the resident uses a commode or bathroom, puts on robe and nonskid footwear. Lowers the bed to its lowest position before the resident gets up.		
17.	Removes and discards gloves. Washes hands.		
18.	Places toilet paper and wipes within resident's reach. Asks resident to clean his hands with a hand wipe when finished if he is able. If resident is using the toilet, asks him not to flush toilet when finished.		
19.	Places call light within resident's reach. Washes hands. Asks resident to signal when finished. Leaves room and closes the door.		
20.	When called by resident, returns and washes hands. Puts on clean gloves.		
21.	Raises bed to safe level. Lowers head of the bed if raised. Makes sure resident is still covered. Does not overexpose the resident. Lowers bed rail on working side if it was raised.		
22.	Removes bedpan carefully. Covers bedpan. Removes and discards bed protector.		
23.	Gives perineal care if help is needed. Wipes from front to back. Dries perineal area with a towel. Helps resident put on undergarment. Covers resident and removes the bath blanket.		

Name: ______________________

24.	Removes and discards bed protector. Places towel in a hamper or bag, and discards disposable supplies.		
25.	Takes bedpan to bathroom. Calls nurse to observe enema results, whether in bedpan or in toilet. Empties contents into toilet.		
26.	Turns the faucet on with a paper towel. Rinses the bedpan with cold water and empties it into the toilet. Flushes toilet. Places bedpan in proper area for cleaning or cleans and stores it according to policy.		
27.	Removes and discards gloves. Washes hands.		
28.	Makes resident comfortable.		
29.	Returns bed to lowest position. Removes privacy measures.		
30.	Leaves call light within resident's reach.		
31.	Washes hands.		
32.	Is courteous and respectful at all times.		
33.	Reports any changes in resident to the nurse. Documents procedure using facility guidelines.		

Date Reviewed ______ Instructor Signature ______

Date Performed ______ Instructor Signature ______

Collecting a stool specimen

		yes	no
1.	Identifies self by name. Identifies resident. Greets resident by name.		
2.	Washes hands.		
3.	Explains procedure to resident. Speaks clearly, slowly, and directly. Maintains face-to-face contact whenever possible.		
4.	Provides for resident's privacy with a curtain, screen, or door.		
5.	Puts on gloves.		
6.	Fits hat to toilet or commode, or provides resident with bedpan.		
7.	When resident is ready to move bowels, asks him not to urinate at the same time. Asks him not to put toilet paper in with sample. Provides a plastic bag for toilet paper.		
8.	Makes sure both bed rails are up, and bed is in its lowest position. Places toilet paper and washcloths or wipes within resident's reach. Asks resident to clean his hands with a hand wipe when finished if he is able.		
9.	Asks resident to signal when he is finished with bowel movement. Makes sure call light is within reach.		
10.	Removes and discards gloves. Washes hands. Leaves room and closes door.		
11.	When called by the resident, returns and washes hands. Puts on clean gloves.		
12.	Gives perineal care if help is needed.		
13.	Using two tongue blades, takes about two tablespoons of stool and puts it in container. Covers it tightly, applies label, and places specimen in a clean biohazard specimen bag. Seals bag.		
14.	Wraps tongue blades in toilet paper and places them in plastic bag with used toilet paper. Discards bag in proper container.		
15.	Turns the faucet on with a paper towel. Rinses the bedpan with cold water and empties it into the toilet. Flushes the toilet. Places bedpan in area for cleaning or cleans and stores it according to policy.		
16.	Removes and discards gloves. Washes hands.		

		yes	no
17.	Makes resident comfortable.		
18.	Returns bed to lowest position. Removes privacy measures.		
19.	Leaves call light within resident's reach.		
20.	Washes hands.		
21.	Is courteous and respectful at all times.		
22.	Reports any changes in resident to the nurse. Documents procedure using facility guidelines. Takes specimen and lab slip to designated place promptly.		

Date Reviewed   Instructor Signature

Date Performed   Instructor Signature

Testing a stool specimen for occult blood

		yes	no
1.	Washes hands.		
2.	Puts on gloves.		
3.	Opens test card.		
4.	Picks up a tongue blade. Gets small amount of stool from specimen container.		
5.	Using a tongue blade, smears a small amount of stool onto Box A of test card.		
6.	Flips tongue blade (or uses new tongue blade). Gets some stool from another part of specimen. Smears small amount of stool onto Box B of test card.		
7.	Closes test card. Turns over to other side.		
8.	Opens flap.		
9.	Opens developer. Applies developer to each box. Follows manufacturer's instructions.		
10.	Waits amount of time listed in instructions, usually between 10 and 60 seconds.		

11.	Watches squares for any color changes. Records color changes. Follows instructions.		
12.	Places tongue blade(s) and test packet in plastic bag.		
13.	Disposes of plastic bag properly in biohazard container.		
14.	Removes and discards gloves.		
15.	Washes hands.		
16.	Documents procedure using facility guidelines. Reports results to the nurse.		

Date Reviewed   Instructor Signature

Date Performed   Instructor Signature

Caring for an ostomy

		yes	no
1.	Identifies self by name. Identifies resident. Greets resident by name.		
2.	Washes hands.		
3.	Explains procedure to resident. Speaks clearly, slowly, and directly. Maintains face-to-face contact whenever possible.		
4.	Provides for resident's privacy with a curtain, screen, or door.		
5.	Adjusts bed to safe working level, usually waist high. Locks bed wheels.		
6.	Puts on gloves.		
7.	Places bed protector under resident. Covers resident with a bath blanket. Pulls down top sheet and blankets. Exposes only ostomy site. Offers resident a towel to keep clothing dry.		
8.	Undoes ostomy belt if used. Pulls on one edge of ostomy pouch to release air.		
9.	Removes ostomy pouch carefully. Places it in plastic bag. Notes color, odor, consistency, and amount of stool in the pouch.		

10.	Wipes area around stoma with disposable wipes for ostomy care. Discards wipes in plastic bag.		
11.	Using a washcloth and warm water, washes area gently in one direction, away from the stoma. Rinses. Pats dry with another towel. Temporarily covers stoma opening with a wipe.		
12.	Applies deodorant to pouch if used. Removes wipe, and places in plastic bag. Puts clean ostomy pouch on resident. Holds in place and seals securely. Makes sure bottom of the pouch is clamped. Attaches to ostomy belt if used.		
13.	Removes bed protector and discards. Places used linens in proper container. Discards plastic bag in proper container.		
14.	Removes and discards gloves. Washes hands.		
15.	Makes resident comfortable.		
16.	Returns bed to lowest position. Removes privacy measures.		
17.	Leaves call light within resident's reach.		
18.	Washes hands.		
19.	Is courteous and respectful at all times.		
20.	Reports any changes in resident to the nurse. Documents procedure using facility guidelines.		

_____   _____
Date Reviewed   Instructor Signature

_____   _____
Date Performed   Instructor Signature

16
The Urinary System

Changing an incontinence brief			
		yes	no
1.	Identifies self by name. Identifies resident. Greets resident by name.		
2.	Washes hands.		
3.	Explains procedure to resident. Speaks clearly, slowly, and directly. Maintains face-to-face contact whenever possible.		
4.	Provides for resident's privacy with a curtain, screen, or door.		
5.	Adjusts bed to safe working level, usually waist high. Raises far bed rail (if used). Locks bed wheels.		
6.	Lowers the head of bed and positions resident flat on her back.		
7.	Covers the resident with a bath blanket		
8.	Puts on gloves.		
9.	Places bed protector under resident.		
10.	Turns resident away from self toward raised bed rail.		
11.	Removes the used incontinence brief, rolling it inward and keeping soiled side inside. Places used brief in the plastic bag without spilling contents.		
12.	Rolls the resident back onto bed protector. Gives perineal care if help is needed.		
13.	Removes and discards gloves. Washes hands. Dons clean gloves.		
14.	Opens tabs on brief. Places brief under resident, centering the back of the pad.		
15.	Wraps brief around resident, making sure front and back of brief cover resident.		

		yes	no
16.	Pulls all tabs to secure the brief. For a male resident, makes sure the penis is placed comfortably.		
17.	Removes and discards bed protector. Covers the resident and removes the bath blanket.		
18.	Removes and discards gloves. Washes hands.		
19.	Makes the resident comfortable.		
20.	Returns bed to lowest position. Leaves bed rails in ordered position. Removes privacy measures.		
21.	Leaves call light within resident's reach.		
22.	Washes hands.		
23.	Is courteous and respectful at all times.		
24.	Reports any changes in resident to the nurse. Documents procedure using facility guidelines.		

_____   _____
Date Reviewed   Instructor Signature

_____   _____
Date Performed   Instructor Signature

Providing catheter care

		yes	no
1.	Identifies self by name. Identifies resident. Greets resident by name.		
2.	Washes hands.		
3.	Explains procedure to resident. Speaks clearly, slowly, and directly. Maintains face-to-face contact whenever possible.		
4.	Provides for resident's privacy with a curtain, screen, or door.		
5.	Adjusts bed to a safe level. Locks bed wheels.		
6.	Lowers head of bed. Positions resident lying flat on her back.		
7.	Removes or folds back top bedding. Keeps resident covered with bath blanket.		

		yes	no
8.	Tests water temperature with thermometer or wrist and ensures it is safe. Has resident check water temperature. Adjusts if necessary.		
9.	Puts on gloves.		
10.	Asks resident to flex her knees and raise buttocks off the bed by pushing against mattress with her feet. Places clean bed protector under her buttocks.		
11.	Exposes only area necessary to clean the catheter.		
12.	Places towel or pad under catheter tubing before washing.		
13.	Wets washcloth and applies soap to washcloth. If a male resident is uncircumcised, pulls back foreskin first. Cleans area around meatus. Uses a clean area of washcloth for each stroke.		
14.	Holds catheter near meatus. Avoids tugging catheter.		
15.	Cleans at least four inches of catheter nearest meatus. Moves in only one direction, away from meatus. Uses a clean area of cloth for each stroke.		
16.	Rinses area around meatus, using a clean area of washcloth for each stroke. Dries area around meatus.		
17.	Rinses at least four inches of catheter nearest meatus. Moves in only one direction, away from meatus. Uses a clean area of the cloth for each stroke.		
18.	Dries at least four inches of the catheter nearest the meatus. Moves in only one direction, away from the meatus. Does not tug catheter.		
19.	Removes and discards bed protector. Removes towel or pad from under catheter tubing and places in proper containers.		

Name: _____

20.	Empties basin in toilet and flushes toilet. Places in proper area for cleaning or cleans and stores it according to facility policy.		
21.	Removes and discards gloves. Washes hands.		
22.	Replaces top covers. Removes bath blanket. Makes resident comfortable.		
23.	Returns bed to lowest position. Removes privacy measures.		
24.	Leaves call light within resident's reach.		
25.	Washes hands.		
26.	Is courteous and respectful at all times.		
27.	Reports any changes in resident to the nurse. Documents procedure using facility guidelines.		

_____   _____
Date Reviewed   Instructor Signature

_____   _____
Date Performed   Instructor Signature

Emptying a catheter drainage bag

		yes	no
1.	Identifies self by name. Identifies resident. Greets resident by name.		
2.	Washes hands.		
3.	Explains procedure to resident. Speaks clearly, slowly, and directly. Maintains face-to-face contact whenever possible.		
4.	Provides for resident's privacy with a curtain, screen, or door.		
5.	Puts on gloves.		
6.	Places graduate on paper towel on the floor.		
7.	Opens drain or clamp on bag. Allows urine to flow out of bag into graduate. Does not let spout or clamp touch graduate.		

8.	When urine has drained, closes clamp. Using alcohol wipe, cleans drain clamp. Returns drain spout to its holder on bag.		
9.	Goes into bathroom. Places graduate on a flat surface and measures at eye level. Notes amount and appearance of urine. Empties urine into toilet and flushes toilet.		
10.	Places container in area for cleaning or cleans and stores it according to policy. Discards paper towel.		
11.	Removes and discards gloves. Washes hands.		
12.	Leaves call light within resident's reach.		
13.	Washes hands.		
14.	Is courteous and respectful at all times.		
15.	Reports any changes in resident to the nurse. Documents procedure and amount of urine (output) using facility guidelines.		

_____   _____
Date Reviewed   Instructor Signature

_____   _____
Date Performed   Instructor Signature

Changing a condom catheter

		yes	no
1.	Identifies self by name. Identifies resident. Greets resident by name.		
2.	Washes hands.		
3.	Explains procedure to resident. Speaks clearly, slowly, and directly. Maintains face-to-face contact whenever possible.		
4.	Provides for resident's privacy with a curtain, screen, or door.		
5.	Adjusts bed to a safe level, usually waist high. Locks bed wheels.		
6.	Lowers head of bed. Positions resident lying flat on his back.		

Name: _____

7.	Removes or folds back top bedding. Keeps resident covered with bath blanket.		
8.	Puts on gloves.		
9.	Places clean bed protector under his buttocks.		
10.	Adjusts bath blanket to expose only genital area.		
11.	Removes condom catheter. Disconnects condom from tube and immediately caps tube. Does not allow tube to touch anything. Places condom and tape in the plastic bag.		
12.	Helps as necessary with perineal care.		
13.	Moves pubic hair away from penis so it does not get rolled into the condom.		
14.	Holds penis firmly. Places condom at tip of penis. Rolls towards base of penis. Leaves at least one inch of space between the drainage tip and glans of penis to prevent irritation. If resident is not circumcised, makes sure that foreskin is in normal position.		
15.	Secures condom to penis with special tape provided. Applies in a spiral. Does not wrap tape all the way around.		
16.	Connects catheter tip to drainage tubing. Does not touch tip to any object but drainage tubing. Makes sure tubing is not twisted or kinked.		
17.	Checks to see if collection bag is secured to leg. Makes sure drain is closed.		
18.	Removes bed protector and discards. Discards plastic bag properly. Places used clothing and linens in proper containers.		
19.	Cleans and stores supplies.		
20.	Removes and discards gloves. Washes hands.		

21.	Replaces top covers. Removes bath blanket. Makes resident comfortable.		
22.	Returns bed to lowest position. Removes privacy measures.		
23.	Leaves call light within resident's reach.		
24.	Washes hands.		
25.	Is courteous and respectful at all times.		
26.	Reports any changes in resident to the nurse. Documents procedure using facility guidelines.		

_____ _____
Date Reviewed   Instructor Signature

_____ _____
Date Performed   Instructor Signature

Collecting a routine urine specimen

		yes	no
1.	Identifies self by name. Identifies resident. Greets resident by name.		
2.	Washes hands.		
3.	Explains procedure to resident. Speaks clearly, slowly, and directly. Maintains face-to-face contact whenever possible.		
4.	Provides for resident's privacy with a curtain, screen, or door.		
5.	Puts on gloves.		
6.	Fits hat to toilet or commode, or provides resident with bedpan or urinal.		
7.	Has resident void into hat, urinal, or bedpan. Asks resident not to put toilet paper or stool in with the sample. Provides a plastic bag to discard toilet paper.		
8.	Makes sure both bed rails are up, and bed is in its lowest position. Places toilet paper and wipes within resident's reach. Asks resident to clean his hands with a hand wipe when finished if he is able.		

9.	Asks resident to signal when he is finished. Makes sure call light is within reach.		
10.	Removes and discards gloves. Washes hands. Leaves room and closes the door.		
11.	When called, returns and washes hands. Puts on clean gloves.		
12.	Gives perineal care if help is needed.		
13.	Takes bedpan, urinal, or commode pail to bathroom.		
14.	Pours urine into specimen container until container is at least half full.		
15.	Covers urine container with its lid. Does not touch inside of container. Wipes off outside with a paper towel and discards. Applies label, and places in clean biohazard specimen bag.		
16.	Discards extra urine in the toilet. Turns the faucet on with a paper towel. Rinses the bedpan, urinal, or hat with cold water and empties it into the toilet. Flushes toilet. Places in proper area for cleaning or cleans it according to policy.		
17.	Removes and discards gloves. Washes hands.		
18.	Makes resident comfortable.		
19.	Returns bed to lowest position. Removes privacy measures.		
20.	Leaves call light within resident's reach.		
21.	Washes hands.		

22.	Is courteous and respectful at all times.		
23.	Reports any changes in resident to the nurse. Documents procedure using facility guidelines. Takes specimen and lab slip to designated place promptly.		

_____   _____
Date Reviewed   Instructor Signature

_____   _____
Date Performed   Instructor Signature

Collecting a clean-catch (midstream) urine specimen

		yes	no
1.	Identifies self by name. Identifies resident. Greets resident by name.		
2.	Washes hands.		
3.	Explains procedure to resident. Speaks clearly, slowly, and directly. Maintains face-to-face contact whenever possible.		
4.	Provides for resident's privacy with a curtain, screen, or door.		
5.	Puts on gloves.		
6.	Opens specimen kit. Does not touch inside of container or lid.		
7.	Cleans perineal area if resident cannot do it.		
8.	Asks resident to urinate a small amount into the bedpan, urinal, or toilet, and to stop before urination is complete.		
9.	Places container under urine stream. Does not touch resident's body with container. Has resident start urinating again. Fills container at least half full. Has resident stop urinating and removes container if possible. Has resident finish urinating in bedpan, urinal, or toilet.		

10.	After urination, gives perineal care if help is needed. Asks resident to clean his hands with hand wipes if he is able.		
11.	Covers urine container with its lid. Does not touch inside of container. Wipes off outside with a paper towel and discards. Applies label, and places in clean biohazard specimen bag.		
12.	Discards extra urine in the toilet. Turns the faucet on with a paper towel. Rinses the bedpan, urinal, or hat with cold water and empties it into the toilet. Flushes toilet. Places in proper area for cleaning or cleans it according to policy.		
13.	Removes and discards gloves. Washes hands.		
14.	Makes resident comfortable.		
15.	Returns bed to lowest position. Removes privacy measures.		
16.	Leaves call light within resident's reach.		
17.	Washes hands.		
18.	Is courteous and respectful at all times.		
19.	Reports any changes in resident to the nurse. Documents procedure using facility guidelines. Takes specimen and lab slip to designated place promptly.		

_____   _____
Date Reviewed   Instructor Signature

_____   _____
Date Performed   Instructor Signature

Collecting a 24-hour urine specimen

		yes	no
1.	Identifies self by name. Identifies resident. Greets resident by name.		
2.	Washes hands.		

3.	Explains procedure to resident. Speaks clearly, slowly, and directly. Maintains face-to-face contact whenever possible. Emphasizes that all urine must be saved. Asks resident not to put toilet paper or stool in with the sample.		
4.	Provides for resident's privacy with a curtain, screen, or door.		
5.	Places a sign near the resident's bed to let all care team members know that a 24-hour specimen is being collected.		
6.	When starting the collection, has resident completely empty the bladder. Measures and notes amount of urine if I&O is being monitored. Discards urine. Notes exact time of this voiding. The collection will run until the same time the next day.		
7.	Washes hands and puts on gloves each time the resident voids.		
8.	Pours urine from bedpan, urinal, or hat into the container. Follows facility policy regarding storing container.		
9.	After each voiding, gives perineal care if help is needed. Asks resident to clean his hands with a hand wipe if he is able.		
10.	After each voiding, places equipment in area for cleaning, or cleans and stores it according to policy.		
11.	Removes and discards gloves.		
12.	Washes hands.		
13.	After the last void of the 24-hour period, adds urine to specimen container. Removes sign.		
14.	Makes resident comfortable.		
15.	Returns bed to lowest position. Removes privacy measures.		
16.	Leaves call light within resident's reach.		

17.	Washes hands.		
18.	Is courteous and respectful at all times.		
19.	Reports any changes in resident to the nurse. Documents procedure using facility guidelines. Takes specimen containers and lab slip to designated place promptly.		

_____   _____
Date Reviewed   Instructor Signature

_____   _____
Date Performed   Instructor Signature

Testing urine with reagent strips

		yes	no
1.	Washes hands.		
2.	Puts on gloves.		
3.	Places paper towel on surface before setting urine specimen down.		
4.	Takes a strip from the bottle and recaps bottle. Closes it tightly.		
5.	Dips strip into specimen.		
6.	Follows manufacturer's instructions for when to remove strip. Removes strip at correct time.		
7.	Follows manufacturer's instructions for how long to wait after removing strip. After proper time has passed, compares strip with color chart on bottle. Does not touch bottle with strip.		
8.	Reads results.		
9.	Stores strips. Discards used items. Discards specimen in the toilet. Flushes toilet.		
10.	Removes and discards gloves.		
11.	Washes hands.		
12.	Records and reports results. Documents procedure using facility guidelines.		

_____   _____
Date Reviewed   Instructor Signature

_____   _____
Date Performed   Instructor Signature

18
The Integumentary System

Applying warm moist compresses

		yes	no
1.	Identifies self by name. Identifies resident. Greets resident by name.		
2.	Washes hands.		
3.	Explains procedure to resident. Speaks clearly, slowly, and directly. Maintains face-to-face contact whenever possible.		
4.	Provides for resident's privacy with a curtain, screen, or door.		
5.	Fills basin one-half to two-thirds with warm water. Tests water temperature with thermometer or wrist. Ensures it is safe. Has resident check water temperature. Adjusts if necessary.		
6.	Soaks washcloth in the water. Wrings it out. Applies it to area needing a warm compress. Notes time. Quickly covers washcloth with plastic wrap and towel to keep it warm.		
7.	Checks area every five minutes. Removes compress if area is red or numb or if resident has pain or discomfort. Changes compress if cooling occurs. Removes compress after 20 minutes.		
8.	Removes privacy measures. Makes resident comfortable.		
9.	Discards plastic wrap. Empties, rinses, and dries basin. Places basin in area for cleaning or cleans and stores it according to policy.		
10.	Places used clothing and linens in appropriate containers.		
11.	Leaves call light within resident's reach.		
12.	Washes hands.		

13.	Is courteous and respectful at all times.		
14.	Reports any changes in resident to the nurse. Documents procedure using facility guidelines.		

_____   _____
Date Reviewed   Instructor Signature

_____   _____
Date Performed   Instructor Signature

Administering warm soaks

		yes	no
1.	Identifies self by name. Identifies resident. Greets resident by name.		
2.	Washes hands.		
3.	Explains procedure to resident. Speaks clearly, slowly, and directly. Maintains face-to-face contact whenever possible.		
4.	Provides for resident's privacy with a curtain, screen, or door.		
5.	Fills basin half full of warm water. Tests water temperature with thermometer or wrist, and ensures it is safe. Has resident check water temperature. Adjusts if necessary.		
6.	Places basin on a disposable absorbent pad (protective barrier), at a comfortable position for the resident.		
7.	Immerses body part in basin. Pads edge of the basin with a towel if needed. Uses a bath blanket to cover resident if needed for extra warmth.		
8.	Checks water temperature every five minutes. Adds warm water as needed to maintain temperature. Observes area for redness. Discontinues soak if resident has pain or discomfort.		
9.	Soaks for 15-20 minutes or as ordered.		
10.	Removes basin. Uses towel to dry resident.		

11.	Removes privacy measures. Makes resident comfortable.		
12.	Empties, rinses, and dries basin. Places basin in area for cleaning or cleans and stores it according to policy.		
13.	Places used clothing and linens in appropriate containers.		
14.	Leaves call light within resident's reach.		
15.	Washes hands.		
16.	Is courteous and respectful at all times.		
17.	Reports any changes in resident to the nurse. Documents procedure using facility guidelines.		

_____   _____
Date Reviewed   Instructor Signature

_____   _____
Date Performed   Instructor Signature

Applying an Aquamatic K-Pad

		yes	no
1.	Identifies self by name. Identifies resident. Greets resident by name.		
2.	Washes hands.		
3.	Explains procedure to resident. Speaks clearly, slowly, and directly. Maintains face-to-face contact whenever possible.		
4.	Provides for resident's privacy with a curtain, screen, or door.		
5.	Makes sure surface on the bedside table is dry. Places control unit on bedside table. Makes sure cords are not frayed or damaged. Checks that tubing between pad and unit is intact.		
6.	Removes cover of control unit to check level of water. If it is low, fills it with distilled water to fill line.		
7.	Puts cover of control unit back in place.		
8.	Plugs unit in. Turns pad on.		

Name: _____

9.	Places pad in the cover. Does not pin pad to cover.		
10.	Uncovers area to be treated. Places covered pad. Notes time. Makes sure tubing is not hanging below bed. Makes sure tubing has no kinks.		
11.	Returns and checks area every five minutes. Removes pad if area is red or numb or if the resident reports pain or discomfort.		
12.	Checks water level. Refills with distilled water to fill line when necessary.		
13.	Turns off unit and removes pad after 20 minutes.		
14.	Removes privacy measures. Makes resident comfortable.		
15.	Cleans and stores supplies.		
16.	Places used linen in appropriate container.		
17.	Leaves call light within resident's reach.		
18.	Washes hands.		
19.	Is courteous and respectful at all times.		
20.	Reports any changes in resident to the nurse. Documents procedure using facility guidelines.		

_____   _____
Date Reviewed   Instructor Signature

_____   _____
Date Performed   Instructor Signature

Assisting with a sitz bath			
		yes	no
1.	Identifies self by name. Identifies resident. Greets resident by name.		
2.	Washes hands.		
3.	Explains procedure to resident. Speaks clearly, slowly, and directly. Maintains face-to-face contact whenever possible.		

4.	Provides for resident's privacy with a curtain, screen, or door.		
5.	Puts on gloves.		
6.	Fills sitz bath container two-thirds full with warm water. Places sitz bath on toilet seat. Checks water temperature using bath thermometer.		
7.	Helps resident undress and get seated on the sitz bath.		
8.	Stays with resident, or leaves the room as ordered. Makes sure resident knows how to use the emergency pull cord in the bathroom if it is needed.		
9.	Helps resident off of the sitz bath after 20 minutes. Provides towels. Helps with dressing if needed.		
10.	Empties and rinses sitz bath container. Discards it properly, according to policy.		
11.	Places used clothing and linens in appropriate containers.		
12.	Removes and discards gloves. Washes hands.		
13.	Makes resident comfortable. Removes privacy measures.		
14.	Leaves call light within resident's reach.		
15.	Washes hands.		
16.	Is courteous and respectful at all times.		
17.	Reports any changes in resident to the nurse. Documents procedure using facility guidelines.		

_____   _____
Date Reviewed   Instructor Signature

_____   _____
Date Performed   Instructor Signature

Name: _____

Applying ice packs

		yes	no
1.	Identifies self by name. Identifies resident. Greets resident by name.		
2.	Washes hands.		
3.	Explains procedure to resident. Speaks clearly, slowly, and directly. Maintains face-to-face contact whenever possible.		
4.	Provides for resident's privacy with a curtain, screen, or door.		
5.	Fills plastic bag or ice pack one-half to two-thirds full with crushed ice. Seals bag. Removes excess air. Covers bag or ice pack with towel or cover.		
6.	Applies pack or bag to the area as ordered. Notes time. Uses another towel to cover bag if it is too cold.		
7.	Checks area after five minutes for blisters or pale, white, or gray skin. Stops treatment if resident reports numbness or pain.		
8.	Removes ice pack or bag after 20 minutes or as ordered.		
9.	Removes privacy measures. Makes resident comfortable.		
10.	Discards supplies or stores in freezer.		
11.	Places used linen in appropriate container.		
12.	Leaves call light within resident's reach.		
13.	Washes hands.		
14.	Is courteous and respectful at all times.		
15.	Reports any changes in resident to the nurse. Documents procedure using facility guidelines.		

_____ _____
Date Reviewed   Instructor Signature

_____ _____
Date Performed   Instructor Signature

Assisting the nurse with changing a nonsterile dressing

		yes	no
1.	Identifies self by name. Identifies resident. Greets resident by name.		
2.	Washes hands.		
3.	Explains procedure to resident. Speaks clearly, slowly, and directly. Maintains face-to-face contact whenever possible.		
4.	Provides for resident's privacy with a curtain, screen, or door.		
5.	Keeps plastic bag close by for disposal of old materials. Cuts pieces of tape long enough to secure the dressing as needed. Opens gauze square packages without touching the insides or the gauze.		
6.	Puts on gloves.		
7.	Only exposes the area where the dressing will be changed. Disposes of used dressing in proper container.		
8.	Removes and discards gloves in plastic bag.		
9.	Washes hands.		
10.	Puts on new gloves. Assists nurse with applying fresh gauze over the wound and taping it in place as needed.		
11.	Removes and discards gloves. Washes hands.		
12.	Makes resident comfortable. Removes privacy measures.		
13.	Leaves call light within resident's reach.		
14.	Washes hands.		

Name: _____

15.	Is courteous and respectful at all times.		
16.	Reports any changes in resident to the nurse. Documents procedure using facility guidelines.		

9.	Keeps gloved hands in front of self and above the level of waist at all times during the procedure.		
10.	Assists nurse with sterile procedure.		

Applying sterile gloves

		yes	no
1.	Washes hands.		
2.	Using a clean, flat, dry surface, removes outer wrapper from gloves. Places inner wrapper on the clean surface. The word *Left* should be on the left side, and the word *Right* should be on the right side.		
3.	Slowly opens the inner wrapper, only touching the small flaps of the wrapper.		
4.	Picks up the first glove by bottom end of the cuff. Slips fingers into the glove without touching the outside of the glove.		
5.	Slips gloved hand into the second glove in the area under the cuff.		
6.	Slowly slips fingers of ungloved hand into the second glove, and pulls it completely over hand and wrist.		
7.	With gloved second hand, finishes pulling first glove up and over the wrist. Adjusts fingers if any adjustment is necessary.		
8.	If either glove has a tear in it, stops and starts again with the second set of sterile gloves.		

19

The Circulatory or Cardiovascular System

Applying knee-high elastic stockings

		yes	no
1.	Identifies self by name. Identifies resident. Greets resident by name.		
2.	Washes hands.		
3.	Explains procedure to resident. Speaks clearly, slowly, and directly. Maintains face-to-face contact whenever possible.		
4.	Provides for resident's privacy with a curtain, screen, or door.		
5.	Adjusts bed to safe working level, usually waist high. Locks bed wheels.		
6.	With resident lying in supine position, removes his socks, shoes, or slippers, and exposes one leg. Exposes no more than one leg at a time.		
7.	Takes one stocking and turns it inside out at least to the heel area.		
8.	Places foot of stocking over toes, foot, and heel. Makes sure heel is in the right place (heel should be in heel of stocking).		
9.	Pulls top of stocking over foot, heel, and leg.		

10.	Makes sure there are no twists or wrinkles in stocking after it is on the leg. Makes sure the heel of the stocking is over the heel of the foot. If the stocking has an opening in the toe area, makes sure the opening is either over or under the toe area.		
11.	Repeats steps 7 through 10 for the other leg.		
12.	Makes resident comfortable.		
13.	Returns bed to lowest position. Removes privacy measures.		
14.	Leaves call light within resident's reach.		
15.	Washes hands.		
16.	Is courteous and respectful at all times.		
17.	Reports any changes in resident to the nurse. Documents procedure using facility guidelines.		

_____   _____
Date Reviewed   Instructor Signature

_____   _____
Date Performed   Instructor Signature

20
The Respiratory System

Collecting a sputum specimen			
		yes	no
1.	Identifies self by name. Identifies resident. Greets resident by name.		
2.	Washes hands.		
3.	Explains procedure to resident. Speaks clearly, slowly, and directly. Maintains face-to-face contact whenever possible.		
4.	Provides for resident's privacy with a curtain, screen, or door.		
5.	Puts on required mask and gloves.		

6.	Asks resident to rinse her mouth with water. Assists as necessary. Has her spit rinse water in the emesis basin if she does not use the sink.		
7.	Stands behind resident and asks her to cough deeply, so that sputum comes up from the lungs. Gives resident tissues to cover her mouth. Asks the resident to spit sputum into container.		
8.	When about two tablespoons of sputum have been obtained, covers container tightly. Wipes any sputum off the outside of the container with tissues. Discards tissues. Applies label and puts container in plastic bag and seals the bag.		
9.	Removes and discards gloves and mask. Washes hands.		
10.	Leaves call light within resident's reach.		
11.	Washes hands.		
12.	Is courteous and respectful at all times.		
13.	Reports any changes in resident to the nurse. Documents procedure using facility guidelines. Takes specimen container and lab slip to the designated place promptly.		

_____   _____
Date Reviewed   Instructor Signature

_____   _____
Date Performed   Instructor Signature

Assisting with deep breathing and coughing exercises			
		yes	no
1.	Identifies self by name. Identifies resident. Greets resident by name.		
2.	Washes hands.		

Name: _____

3.	Explains procedure to resident. Speaks clearly, slowly, and directly. Maintains face-to-face contact whenever possible.		
4.	Provides for resident's privacy with a curtain, screen, or door.		
5.	Puts on gloves.		
6.	Positions resident in Fowler's position with a pillow over abdomen if needed.		
7.	Asks her to wrap her arms around the pillow and hold pillow tightly against her abdomen.		
8.	Tells resident to take a deep breath and hold the breath for a few seconds.		
9.	Asks the resident to exhale for as long as possible through lips that are pursed.		
10.	Tells resident to then repeat the deep breathing exercise a few more times.		
11.	Makes sure tissues are nearby. Asks resident to hold the pillow tightly, breathe in once deeply, and then cough as forcefully as possible. Collects any secretions with the tissues and disposes of tissues temporarily in the emesis basin.		
12.	Repeats sequence above the designated number of times.		
13.	Disposes of tissues in nearest no-touch receptacle.		
14.	Empties, rinses, and dries basin. Places basin in designated dirty supply area or returns to storage, depending on facility policy.		
15.	Removes and discards gloves. Washes hands.		
16.	Makes resident comfortable. Removes privacy measures.		
17.	Leaves call light within resident's reach.		
18.	Washes hands.		

19.	Is courteous and respectful at all times.		
20.	Reports any changes in resident to the nurse. Documents procedure using facility guidelines.		

Date Reviewed _____ Instructor Signature _____

Date Performed _____ Instructor Signature _____

Assisting with an incentive spirometer

		yes	no
1.	Identifies self by name. Identifies resident. Greets resident by name.		
2.	Washes hands.		
3.	Explains procedure to resident. Speaks clearly, slowly, and directly. Maintains face-to-face contact whenever possible.		
4.	Provides for resident's privacy with a curtain, screen, or door.		
5.	Adjusts bed to a safe level, usually waist high. Locks bed wheels.		
6.	Positions resident sitting upright in bed or chair.		
7.	Puts on gloves.		
8.	Cleans mouthpiece as directed.		
9.	Slides indicator to correct level as indicated in care plan.		
10.	Asks resident to grasp the spirometer and exhale fully.		
11.	Asks resident to wrap his lips around the mouthpiece and inhale slowly and deeply.		
12.	Asks resident to keep the indicator at the designated level for as long as possible. Lets resident know to exhale once he cannot keep the indicator at the designated level.		
13.	Repeats steps as ordered in care plan. Stops the procedure if the resident becomes dizzy.		

		yes	no
14.	Places the spirometer in the correct area for cleaning or cleans and stores according to policy.		
15.	Removes and discards gloves.		
16.	Returns bed to lowest position. Makes resident comfortable. Removes privacy measures.		
17.	Leaves call light within resident's reach.		
18.	Washes hands.		
19.	Is courteous and respectful at all times.		
20.	Reports any changes in resident to the nurse. Documents procedure using facility guidelines.		

Date Reviewed _____ Instructor Signature _____

Date Performed _____ Instructor Signature _____

		yes	no
9.	Assists resident to replace eyeglasses on face. Places over the ears and positions comfortably.		
10.	Makes resident comfortable. Removes privacy measures.		
11.	Leaves call light within resident's reach.		
12.	Washes hands.		
13.	Is courteous and respectful at all times.		
14.	Reports any changes in resident to the nurse. Documents procedure using facility guidelines.		

Date Reviewed _____ Instructor Signature _____

Date Performed _____ Instructor Signature _____

22
The Nervous System

Caring for eyeglasses			
		yes	no
1.	Identifies self by name. Identifies resident. Greets resident by name.		
2.	Washes hands.		
3.	Explains procedure to resident. Speaks clearly, slowly, and directly. Maintains face-to-face contact whenever possible.		
4.	Provides for resident's privacy with a curtain, screen, or door.		
5.	Removes eyeglasses and places in emesis basin.		
6.	Lines sink with towel.		
7.	Cleans eyeglasses over lined sink with proper solution and lens cloth		
8.	Dries with soft, 100% cotton cloth or special lens cloth. Does not dry with tissues, as they may scratch eyeglasses.		

23
The Endocrine System

Providing foot care for a resident with diabetes			
		yes	no
1	Identifies self by name. Identifies resident. Greets resident by name.		
2.	Washes hands.		
3.	Explains procedure to resident. Speaks clearly, slowly, and directly. Maintains face-to-face contact whenever possible.		
4.	Provides for resident's privacy with a curtain, screen, or door.		
5.	If the resident is in bed, adjusts bed to lowest position. Locks bed wheels.		
6.	Fills basin halfway with warm water. Tests water temperature with thermometer or wrist. Ensures it is safe. Has resident check water temperature. Adjusts if necessary.		
7.	Places basin on a disposable absorbent pad (protective barrier). Supports foot and ankle throughout procedure.		

Name: _____

8.	Puts on gloves.		
9.	Removes resident's socks. Completely submerges resident's feet in water. Soaks feet for 10 to 20 minutes.		
10.	Removes one foot from water. Washes entire foot, including between the toes and around nail beds, with a soapy washcloth.		
11.	Rinses entire foot, including between the toes.		
12.	Using a towel, pats dry entire foot, including between the toes.		
13.	Repeats steps 10 through 12 for the other foot.		
14.	Puts lotion in hand. Warms lotion by rubbing hands together.		
15.	Starting at the toes and working up to the ankles, rubs lotion into the feet with circular strokes. Does not put lotion between the toes. Removes excess lotion with a towel. Makes sure lotion has been absorbed and feet are completely dry.		
16.	Observes feet, ankles, and legs carefully, checking for things like dry skin, skin tears, red areas, corns, blisters, calluses, warts, rashes, or bruises.		
17.	Helps resident put on clean socks and shoes or slippers.		
18.	Empties, rinses, and dries basin. Places basin in designated dirty supply area or returns to storage, depending on facility policy.		
19.	Places used linen in the proper container.		
20.	Removes and discards gloves. Washes hands.		
21.	Makes resident comfortable.		

22.	Removes privacy measures.		
23.	Leaves call light within resident's reach.		
24.	Washes hands.		
25.	Is courteous and respectful at all times.		
26.	Reports any changes in resident to the nurse. Documents procedure using facility guidelines.		

_____   _____
Date Reviewed   Instructor Signature

_____   _____
Date Performed   Instructor Signature

25
Rehabilitation and Restorative Care

Assisting with ambulation for a resident using a cane, walker, or crutches			
		yes	no
1.	Identifies self by name. Identifies resident. Greets resident by name.		
2.	Washes hands.		
3.	Explains procedure to resident. Speaks clearly, slowly, and directly. Maintains face-to-face contact whenever possible.		
4.	Provides for resident's privacy with a curtain, screen, or door.		
5.	Adjusts bed to lowest position. Locks bed wheels. Assists resident to sitting position so that resident's feet are flat on the floor.		
6.	Puts nonskid footwear on resident and securely fastens.		
7.	Stands with feet about shoulder-width apart. Bends knees. Keeps back straight.		

8.	Places transfer belt around resident's waist over clothing (not on bare skin). Checks to make sure that skin or skin folds (for example, breasts) are not caught under the belt. Grasps belt securely on both sides, with hands in an upward position.		
9.	If resident is unable to stand without help, braces (supports) resident's lower extremities.		
10.	On three, with hands still grasping the transfer belt on both sides and moving upward, slowly helps resident to stand.		
11.	Helps as needed with ambulation with cane, walker, or crutches.		
12.	Walks slightly behind and on the weaker side of resident while holding onto the transfer belt.		
13.	Watches for obstacles in the resident's path. Asks resident to look ahead, not down at his feet.		
14.	Encourages resident to rest if he is tired. Lets resident set the pace. Discusses how far he plans to go based on care plan.		
15.	After ambulation, removes transfer belt. Makes resident comfortable.		
16.	Leaves bed in lowest position. Removes privacy measures.		
17.	Leaves call light within resident's reach.		
18.	Washes hands.		
19.	Is courteous and respectful at all times.		
20.	Reports any changes in resident to the nurse. Documents procedure using facility guidelines.		

_____ _____
Date Reviewed   Instructor Signature

_____ _____
Date Performed   Instructor Signature

Assisting with passive range of motion exercises

		yes	no
1.	Identifies self by name. Identifies resident. Greets resident by name.		
2.	Washes hands.		
3.	Explains procedure to resident. Speaks clearly, slowly, and directly. Maintains face-to-face contact whenever possible.		
4.	Provides for resident's privacy with a curtain, screen, or door.		
5.	Adjusts bed to a safe level, usually waist high. Locks bed wheels.		
6.	Positions resident lying supine on the bed. Positions body in proper alignment.		
7.	While supporting the limbs, moves all joints gently, slowly, and smoothly through the range of motion to the point of resistance. Repeats each exercise at least three times. Stops exercises if any pain occurs.		
8.	*Shoulder*		
	Performs the following movements properly, supporting the resident's arm at the elbow and wrist by placing one hand under the elbow and the other hand under the wrist:		
	1. Extension		
	2. Flexion		
	3. Abduction		
	4. Adduction		
9.	*Elbow*		
	Performs the following movements properly, holding the wrist with one hand, and holding the elbow with the other:		
	1. Flexion		
	2. Extension		
	3. Pronation		
	4. Supination		

10.	*Wrist*		
	Performs the following movements properly, holding the wrist with one hand, and using the fingers of the other hand to help the joint through the motions:		
	1. Flexion		
	2. Dorsiflexion		
	3. Radial flexion		
	4. Ulnar flexion		
11.	*Thumb*		
	Performs the following movements properly:		
	1. Abduction		
	2. Adduction		
	3. Opposition		
	4. Flexion		
	5. Extension		
12.	*Fingers*		
	Performs the following movements properly:		
	1. Flexion		
	2. Extension		
	3. Abduction		
	4. Adduction		
13.	*Hip*		
	Performs the following movements properly, placing one hand under the knee and one under the ankle:		
	1. Abduction		
	2. Adduction		
	3. Internal rotation		
	4. External rotation		
14.	*Knees*		
	Performs the following movements properly, placing one hand under the knee and one under the ankle:		
	1. Flexion		
	2. Extension		

15.	*Ankles*		
	Performs the following movements properly, supporting the foot and ankle:		
	1. Dorsiflexion		
	2. Plantar flexion		
	3. Supination		
	4. Pronation		
16.	*Toes*		
	Performs the following movements properly:		
	1. Flexion		
	2. Extension		
	3. Abduction		
17.	Returns bed to lowest position. Removes privacy measures.		
18.	Leaves call light within resident's reach.		
19.	Washes hands.		
20.	Is courteous and respectful at all times.		
21.	Reports any changes in resident to the nurse. Documents procedure using facility guidelines.		

Date Reviewed _____ Instructor Signature _____

Date Performed _____ Instructor Signature _____

26
Subacute Care

Applying a pulse oximetry device			
		yes	no
1.	Identifies self by name. Identifies resident. Greets resident by name.		
2.	Washes hands.		
3.	Explains procedure to resident. Speaks clearly, slowly, and directly. Maintains face-to-face contact whenever possible.		
4.	Provides for resident's privacy with a curtain, screen, or door.		

5.	Cleans finger or body area where sensor will be placed using cleansing wipe.		
6.	Removes sensor from package and places on finger, toe, or earlobe. Ensures it is on correctly.		
7.	Turns on the device. The pulse oximetry reading should appear on the screen quickly.		
8.	Asks resident to not remove or adjust pulse oximetry device. Asks resident to press call signal if the device comes off or dislodges.		
9.	Makes resident comfortable.		
10.	Removes privacy measures.		
11.	Leaves call light within resident's reach.		
12.	Washes hands.		
13.	Is courteous and respectful at all times.		
14.	Reports any changes in resident to the nurse. Documents procedure using facility guidelines.		

_____   _____
Date Reviewed   Instructor Signature

_____   _____
Date Performed   Instructor Signature

27
End-of-Life Care

Postmortem care			
		yes	no
1.	Identifies resident.		
2.	Washes hands.		
3.	Explains procedure to resident's family and asks them to step outside. Is courteous, respectful, and compassionate at all times.		
4.	Provides for privacy with a curtain, screen, or door.		
5.	Adjusts bed to safe working level, usually waist high. Locks bed wheels.		

6.	Avoids trauma to the resident's body throughout the procedure. Treats body with utmost respect.		
7.	Puts on gloves.		
8.	Turns off any oxygen, suction, or other equipment, if directed by the nurse. Does not remove any tubes or other equipment.		
9.	Closes eyes without pressure.		
10.	Positions body in good alignment, on the back with legs straight. Folds arms across the abdomen.		
11.	Closes mouth. Places rolled towel under the chin.		
12.	Gently bathes body. Is careful to avoid bruising. Replaces any dressings only if directed to do so.		
13.	Combs or brushes hair gently without tugging.		
14.	Places drainage pads where needed, usually under the head and/or under the perineal area and buttocks.		
15.	Puts a clean gown on the body.		
16.	Covers body to just over the shoulders with sheet. Does not cover face or head.		
17.	Tidies room so family may visit.		
18.	Removes all used supplies and linen.		
19.	Follows facility policy for handling or removing personal items.		
20.	Removes and discards gloves.		
21.	Washes hands.		
22.	Returns bed to low position if raised. Turns lights down and allows family to enter and spend private time with resident.		
23.	Returns after family departs and puts on clean gloves.		
24.	Places shroud on resident and follows instructions on completing ID tags.		

Name: _____

25.	Removes and discards gloves.		
26.	Washes hands.		
27.	Reports and records observations. Documents procedure using facility guidelines.		

_____   _____
Date Reviewed   Instructor Signature

_____   _____
Date Performed   Instructor Signature

Practice Exam

After a nursing assistant has completed an approved training program in her state, she is given a competency evaluation (a certification exam or test) in order to be certified to work in that state. This exam usually consists of both a written evaluation and a skills evaluation. Review the guidelines for taking exams located in the appendix of the textbook on page 508.

1. One task commonly assigned to nursing assistants is
    (A) Inserting and removing tubes
    (B) Changing sterile dressings
    (C) Helping residents with elimination needs
    (D) Prescribing medications to residents

2. When a resident refuses to let the nursing assistant measure her blood pressure, the nursing assistant should
    (A) Tell the resident that she must have it taken to prevent a serious illness
    (B) Take the resident's blood pressure anyway and report the refusal later
    (C) Tell the resident that if she does this, she will get her dinner tray delivered earlier
    (D) Report this to the nurse

3. If a nursing assistant suspects that a resident is being abused, he should
    (A) Report it to the nurse immediately
    (B) Confront the abuser
    (C) Keep watching until he is sure abuse is occurring
    (D) Call the resident's family immediately to report the possible abuse

4. One safety device that helps transfer residents is called a
    (A) Waist restraint
    (B) Posey vest
    (C) Transfer belt
    (D) Geriatric chair

5. A nursing assistant may share a resident's medical information with which of the following?
    (A) The resident's friends
    (B) Other members of the healthcare team
    (C) The nursing assistant's friends
    (D) The resident's roommate

6. Which of the following is an objective statement?
    (A) Mr. Harris has a rash on his back.
    (B) Mrs. Carpenter has been having headaches lately.
    (C) Mr. Jansson says his medication makes him nauseous.
    (D) Ms. McDowell's knees hurt when she is walking.

7. When may a nursing assistant hit a resident?
    (A) When the resident becomes combative
    (B) When the resident threatens to hit the nursing assistant or someone else
    (C) Only if the resident hits the nursing assistant first
    (D) Never

8. When giving perineal care to a female resident, a nursing assistant should
    (A) Wipe from front to back
    (B) Wipe from back to front
    (C) Use the same section of the washcloth for cleaning each part
    (D) Wash the anal area before the perineal area

9. How many milliliters (mL) equal one ounce?
    (A) 40
    (B) 30
    (C) 60
    (D) 20

10. According to OBRA, nursing assistants must complete at least ___ hours of training and must pass a competency evaluation before they can be employed.
    (A) 100
    (B) 250
    (C) 50
    (D) 75

11. Call lights should be placed
    (A) On the wall over the head of the bed
    (B) Inside the bedside stand
    (C) On the floor
    (D) Within the resident's reach

12. An ombudsman is a person who
    (A) Is in charge of hiring facility staff
    (B) Teaches nursing assistants how to perform range of motion exercises
    (C) Is a legal advocate for residents and helps protect their rights
    (D) Creates special diets for residents who are ill

13. To best communicate with a resident who has a hearing impairment, the nursing assistant should
    (A) Use short sentences and simple words
    (B) Shout the words slowly
    (C) Approach the resident from behind
    (D) Raise the pitch of her voice

14. Which temperature site is considered the most accurate?
    (A) Rectum (rectal)
    (B) Mouth (oral)
    (C) Armpit (axillary)
    (D) Ear (tympanic)

15. Psychosocial needs include
    (A) Need for activity
    (B) Need for sleep and rest
    (C) Need for love and acceptance
    (D) Need for clothing and shelter

16. How should a standard bedpan be positioned?
    (A) It should be positioned however the resident prefers.
    (B) The wider end should be aligned with the resident's buttocks.
    (C) The smaller end should be aligned with the resident's buttocks.
    (D) The smaller end should be facing the resident's head.

17. If a nursing assistant encounters a sexual situation between two consenting adult residents, he should
    (A) Provide privacy
    (B) Ask the residents to stop
    (C) Discuss it with a clergyperson
    (D) Tell other residents

18. The single most important thing a nursing assistant can do to prevent the spread of disease is to
    (A) Wear a waterproof watch
    (B) Wash her hands
    (C) Apply and use personal protective equipment correctly
    (D) Practice Transmission-Based Precautions on every resident

19. If a resident has diabetes, what should a nursing assistant do with regard to the resident's toenails?
    (A) Never cut them
    (B) Cut them when the resident requests it
    (C) Cut them weekly
    (D) File them into rounded edges

20. Most of the accidents in a facility are related to
    (A) Burns and scalds
    (B) Failing to identify residents before performing care
    (C) Choking
    (D) Falls

21. When a resident has right-sided weakness, how should clothing be applied first?
    (A) On the left side
    (B) On the right side
    (C) On whichever side is closer to the nursing assistant
    (D) On whichever side the resident prefers

22. One way a nursing assistant can help a new resident adjust to life in a facility is to
    (A) Tell the resident how much work it is to care for him
    (B) Hide any mistakes the nursing assistant makes so that the resident will feel more confident in her work
    (C) Listen if the resident wants to express his feelings
    (D) Push the resident to join in activities even if he does not want to because it is the best thing for him

23. In what order should the nursing assistant perform range of motion exercises?
    (A) Start from the feet and work up
    (B) Start from the shoulders and work down
    (C) Exercise the arms and legs first
    (D) Exercise the arms and legs last

24. A bed made while the resident is in the bed is called a(n)
    (A) Open bed
    (B) Closed bed
    (C) Occupied bed
    (D) Surgical bed

25. When providing personal care, the nursing assistant should
    (A) Do the task for the resident if it seems like it will take him a long time to complete it
    (B) Provide privacy for the resident
    (C) Tell the resident about other residents' conditions to distract him
    (D) Discuss her personal problems to get the resident's advice

26. Observing for changes in residents' skin is especially important to help prevent
    (A) Falls
    (B) Pressure injuries
    (C) Edema
    (D) Weight gain

27. Generally speaking, the last sense to leave a dying person is the sense of
    (A) Sight
    (B) Taste
    (C) Smell
    (D) Hearing

28. If a nursing assistant cannot obtain a reading when measuring vital signs, she should
    (A) Record her best guess
    (B) Use the previous reading for that resident
    (C) Leave that space in the chart blank
    (D) Tell the nurse

29. When donning personal protective equipment, which of the following should be donned (put on) first?
    (A) Mask
    (B) Gown
    (C) Gloves
    (D) Goggles

30. According to the USDA's MyPlate, which food groups should make up the largest proportion of the diet?
    (A) Vegetables and fruits
    (B) Proteins and grains
    (C) Grains and fruits
    (D) Dairy products and proteins

31. The process of helping to restore a person to the highest level of functioning is called
    (A) Positioning
    (B) Rehabilitation
    (C) Elimination
    (D) Retention

32. To prevent dehydration, a nursing assistant should
    (A) Discourage fluids before bedtime
    (B) Withhold fluids so the resident will be really thirsty
    (C) Offer fresh water and other fluids often
    (D) Wake the resident during the night to offer fluids

33. A resident tells a nursing assistant that she is scared of dying. Which of the following would be the best response from the nursing assistant?
    (A) The NA can offer to call her minister to see if he can visit the resident.
    (B) The NA can listen quietly and ask questions when appropriate.
    (C) The NA can reassure the resident that she is not dying soon.
    (D) The NA can suggest other medications that might help with the resident's condition.

34. Regarding catheters, it is important for a nursing assistant to remember that
    (A) Tubing should be kinked to work properly
    (B) Perineal care does not need to be performed
    (C) The drainage bag should be kept lower than the hips or the bladder
    (D) The resident should lie on top of the tubing

35. Which of the following would be the best response if a nursing assistant sees a resident masturbating?
    (A) The NA should ask the charge nurse what she is legally allowed to do.
    (B) The NA should provide privacy for the resident.
    (C) The NA should suggest that nighttime might be better for masturbating.
    (D) The NA should ask the resident to stop masturbating.

36. One way for a nursing assistant to promote normal urination is to
    (A) Reduce residents' intake of fluids
    (B) Discourage activity and exercise
    (C) Provide plenty of privacy and time for elimination
    (D) Ask residents to wait as long as they can before urinating so as to train the bladder to hold more fluids

37. When assisting a resident who has had a stroke, a nursing assistant should
    (A) Do everything for the resident
    (B) Lead with the stronger side when transferring
    (C) Dress the stronger side first
    (D) Place food in the weaker side of the mouth

38. In which stage would a dying resident be if he insists that a mistake was made on his blood test and he is not really dying?
    (A) Denial
    (B) Bargaining
    (C) Acceptance
    (D) Depression

39. When should elastic stockings be applied?
    (A) In the morning
    (B) In the afternoon
    (C) Right before bedtime
    (D) Just after lunch

40. How should dentures be stored after they are cleaned?
    (A) In a labeled denture cup
    (B) On a paper towel on the overbed table
    (C) In the sink in the resident's bathroom
    (D) In tissues on the resident's bedside stand

41. When lifting an object, a nursing assistant can use proper body mechanics by
    (A) Holding the object away from his body
    (B) Keeping both of his feet close together
    (C) Lifting with the muscles in his lower back
    (D) Bending his knees and keeping his back straight

42. To best respond to a resident with Alzheimer's disease who is repeating a question over and over again, the nursing assistant should
    (A) Answer the question each time it is asked, using the same words
    (B) Try to silence the resident
    (C) Ask the resident to stop repeating herself
    (D) Explain to the resident that she just asked that question

43. To locate the radial pulse, the nursing assistant should place her fingertips on the resident's
    (A) Neck
    (B) Wrist
    (C) Chest
    (D) Foot

44. When providing ostomy care, which of the following should the nursing assistant do first?
    (A) Undo the ostomy belt
    (B) Remove the ostomy pouch
    (C) Wash her hands
    (D) Place a bed protector under the resident

45. When performing mouth care for a resident who is unconscious, in which position should the nursing assistant place the resident?
(A) On his back (supine)
(B) On his side (lateral)
(C) On his stomach (prone)
(D) On his stomach with his knees pulled up toward the abdomen and the legs separated (knee-chest)

46. Which of the following is the safest type of razor to use?
(A) Electric razor
(B) Safety razor
(C) Disposable razor
(D) Steel razor

47. A nursing assistant must wear gloves when
(A) Combing a resident's hair
(B) Feeding a resident
(C) Performing mouth care
(D) Performing range of motion exercises

48. To best communicate with a resident who has a vision impairment, the nursing assistant should
(A) Rearrange furniture without telling the resident
(B) Identify herself when she enters the room
(C) Keep the lighting low at all times
(D) Touch the resident before identifying herself

49. Skin breakdown usually occurs at areas of the body that bear the greatest amount of weight, called
(A) Integuments
(B) Deep tissues
(C) Pressure points
(D) Necrosis

50. How should soiled bed linens be handled?
(A) By carrying them away from the nursing assistant's body
(B) By shaking them in the air to get rid of contaminants
(C) By taking them into another resident's room to put them in a hamper
(D) By rolling them dirty side out

Name: _____